Scotland's Contribution to Naval and Military Medicine and Surgery

How doctors trained in Scotland enhanced its progress from the 18th century to the First World War

Edited by
Iain Macintyre, Hilary Morris, Andreas K Demetriades

Helion & Company

Helion & Company Limited
Unit 8 Amherst Business Centre
Budbrooke Road
Warwick
CV34 5WE
England
Tel. 01926 499619
Email: info@helion.co.uk
Website: www.helion.co.uk
X (formerly Twitter): @Helionbooks
Facebook: @HelionBooks
Visit our blog at https://helionbooks.wordpress.com/

Published by Helion & Company 2024
Designed and typeset by Mach 3 Solutions (www.mach3solutions.co.uk)
Cover designed by Paul Hewitt, Battlefield Design (www.battlefield-design.co.uk)

ISBN 978-1-804516-26-3

British Library Cataloguing-in-Publication Data.
A catalogue record for this book is available from the British Library.

Contents

List of Illustrations

Chapter 3

Chapter 4

Chapter 5

Chapter 6

Chapter 11

Chapter 12

Introduction

Scotland's reputation for medical education is a long-standing one, so that both the number and the influence of doctors trained in Scotland have been out of all proportion to the size of the country or its population.

The reasons for this are not hard to find. The surgeons and barbers of Edinburgh were required, by the terms of their 1505 charter, to be able to read and to write Latin, unusual if not unique requirements for a medieval craft incorporation. These conditions could be seen as the start of a tradition of medical education in Scotland. At the end of the sixteenth century the Faculty of Physicians and Surgeons of Glasgow was founded by Peter Lowe, who had practised as a military surgeon in France before returning to his native Scotland. But it was the foundation of the Edinburgh University medical school in 1726 that would lead to Scotland emerging as a leader in world medical education. A leading light in the establishment of this medical school was another military surgeon, John Monro, founder of the Monro medical dynasty who would help enhance the city's reputation for medical teaching over the generations. Based on the Leiden model, where many of its teachers had trained, the Edinburgh Medical School was the first in the British Isles to offer university teaching linked to a teaching hospital and leading to a medical degree. The new school attracted students from all over the world, drawn both by the quality of the teaching (which was largely in English) and by the prestige of the Edinburgh MD degree. Such was demand that a flourishing extramural school grew up around the university. In the early eighteenth century Glasgow University had begun to examine for the MD degree, and as the city of Glasgow grew and flourished so too did its medical school, and, as in Edinburgh, an extramural school developed.

In Aberdeen a 'mediciner' had been on the university staff since 1495 making it the oldest chair in Britain for the teaching of medicine and its two ancient university colleges, Kings and Marischal College both conferred medical degrees. It was not until the Medical Act of 1858 that these were united and an undergraduate medical school was formally established. St Andrews University too offered medical degrees, although until the early nineteenth century many of these were of dubious provenance and quality.

In this context it is easy to understand Charles Newman's quite remarkable statistic that between 1800 and 1850 some 96 percent of doctors in Britain with a medical degree had received their medical education in Scotland.[1]

Throughout the eighteenth century and for most of the nineteenth century, Scotland produced more medical graduates than could find gainful employment in Scotland or even in Britain. The expanding empire, and the armed forces required to defend it, needed doctors and it was inevitable that Scottish medical graduates should come to be over-represented in the medical services of the British Army and the Royal Navy. Kaufman calculated that of the 837 army medical officers with a university degree between 1806 and 1856, no fewer than 697 (83.2 percent) had received that degree from a Scottish university.[2]

There were other qualifications which attracted potential military medics to Scotland. From 1778, the Royal College of Surgeons of Edinburgh offered a new diploma which qualified the holder to act as a surgeons' mate in the armed forces. In the face of inevitable opposition from London, these were accepted by the relevant Army and Navy Boards and, from 1805, these diplomas became accepted as qualification for assistant surgeons in the Army and shortly after accepted as an entry qualification for Army surgeons.[3]

In recognition of this tradition, the Scottish Society of the History of Medicine and the History of Medicine Society of the Royal Society of Medicine hosted an online symposium in 2023 to present a series of lectures under the title, 'Scotland's Contribution to Naval and Military Medicine.'

Each of the chapters in this volume is based on a presentation to that symposium. These highlight individuals and events which together add to our knowledge about some of the many contributions to naval and military medicine made by Scottish medical graduates between the eighteenth century and the First World War.

Publication of this book was made possible by generous financial support from the Douglas Guthrie Trust.

Iain Macintyre
Hilary Morris
Andreas K. Demetriades
September 2024

1 Charles Newman in F. N. L. Poynter (ed.), *The Evolution of Medical Education in Britain* (London, Pitman Medical, 1966) p.49.

2 Matthew Kaufman, *Surgeons at War. Medical Arrangements for the Treatment of the Sick and Wounded in the British Army During the Late 18th and 19th Centuries* (London, Greenwood Press, 2001), pp.111–112.

3 Matthew Kaufman, *Medical Teaching in Edinburgh During the 18th and 19th Centuries.* (Edinburgh, Royal College of Surgeons of Edinburgh, 2003), pp.9–10.

Bibliography

Kaufman, Matthew *Medical Teaching in Edinburgh During the 18th and 19th Centuries.* (Edinburgh, Royal College of Surgeons of Edinburgh, 2003) pp.9–10

Kaufman, Matthew, *Surgeons at War. Medical Arrangements for the Treatment of the Sick and Wounded in the British Army During the Late 18th and 19th Centuries* (London, Greenwood Press, 2001) pp.111–112

Newman, Charles in F. N. L. Poynter (ed.), *The Evolution of Medical Education in Britain* (London, Pitman Medical, 1966), p.49

1

Bringing Enlightenment Thinking to the Battlefield; Sir John Pringle's *Observations on the Diseases of the Army*

Iain Macintyre

Sir John Pringle (1707–1782) had a remarkably varied career as physician, professor of philosophy, laboratory scientist, military Physician General and royal physician. His philosopher's approach, combined with a gift for astute observation, enabled him to apply Enlightenment thinking to medical ailments in the Army, both during his army career as Physician General and for decades afterwards through the medium of his highly influential book, *Observations on the Diseases of the Army*. The conclusions that he drew proved to be an early contribution to germ theory and furthered the later understanding of the cause of communicable disease and of its prevention. *Observations* became a stimulus and a template for later books on military medicine and Pringle came to be regarded as the founder of British military medicine.

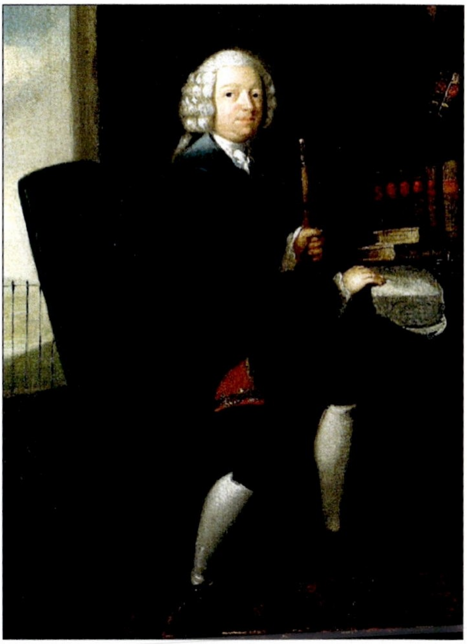

Sir John Pringle. Unknown artist. (Wellcome Collection. Public Domain)

Pringle's Education

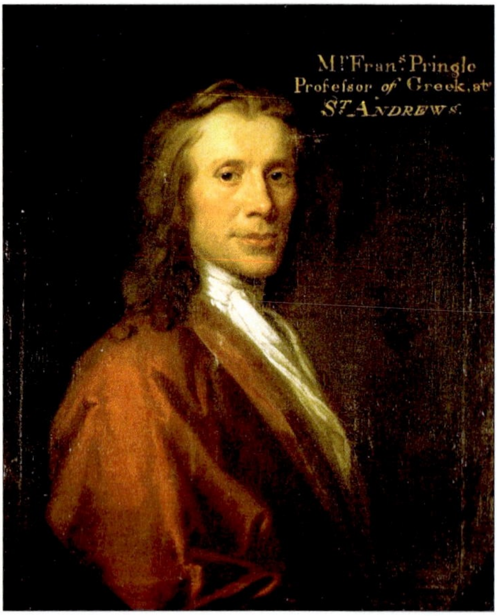

Francis Pringle, Professor of Greek, St Andrews University. Portrait attributed to William Aikman. (University of St Andrews Libraries and Museums, ID: HC217)

Pringle was the youngest son of Sir John Pringle (1662–1721), 2nd Baronet of Stichill, near Kelso in the Scottish Borders.[1] His education was crucial in enabling him to make the observations and to formulate the hypotheses which he applied to the diseases he later observed in the army.

He studied philosophy and classics at the University of St Andrews, taught in part by his father's cousin Francis Pringle (*c.* 1665–1752), Professor of Philosophy and Greek at St Leonard's College. At St Andrews he was introduced to philosophical concepts that were to become a feature of the Scottish Enlightenment, including inquiry, experiment and utility – the concept that acquired knowledge should be used for the common good.

Pringle's fifth year was devoted to the study of the works of the philosopher Francis Bacon (1561–1626) which was to influence his thinking throughout his professional life.[2] Bacon had introduced inductive reasoning, a process which involved making and recording observations, reasoning from these to formulate hypotheses which were then tested with further observation, reading or experiment.

His medical education began in 1727 at the University of Edinburgh's recently founded medical school, where he came under the influence of the physician and philosopher George Young (1692–1757), an empiric who emphasised observation, practical experience and a sceptical approach to evidence in medicine.[3] Pringle readily espoused this doctrine which he continued to practice throughout his career. Young was a disciple of Thomas Sydenham (1624–1689) and Pringle too would adopt Sydenham's philosophy of closely observing the patients and recording their clinical features. Like Young, Pringle became a member of the Rankenian Club, an influential

1 Andrew Kippis, *Six Discourses, delivered by Sir John Pringle, Bart.: To Which is Prefixed a Life of the Author*, (London: Strahan and T. Cadell, 1783).

2 Morris McCrae, *Saving the Army. The life of Sir John Pringle*. (Edinburgh: Birlinn, 2014), p.12.

3 Iain Macintyre, 'A sceptic and an Empiric in Medicine: George Young (1692–1757) and the Beginnings of the Scottish Medical Enlightenment' in *Journal of the Royal College of Physicians of Edinburgh*, 42:4 (2012), pp.352–360. http://dx.doi.org/10.4997/JRCPE.2012.415 (accessed 14 October 2023)

philosophy club whose members included many self-styled 'literati', leaders of the Scottish Enlightenment.[4] His uncle Dr Francis Pringle, who was President of the Royal College of Physicians of Edinburgh from 1727 to 1731, probably influenced his decision to become a physician.

To further this ambition John Pringle then went to Leiden, the leading medical school of the day. Here he studied under Herman Boerhaave (1668–1738) from whom he learned the theory of iatro-mechanical medicine, the concept that many bodily functions could be better explained by mechanical forces rather than imbalance of humors. Despite this innovative teaching and for all his scepticism and rational thinking, Pringle continued to practice humoral medicine throughout his career. In Leiden Boerhaave had started clinical bedside teaching which placed further emphasis on clinical observation and on Baconian inductive reasoning. Pringle graduated from the University of Leiden in 1730, dedicating his doctoral thesis to the two relatives who had most influenced his career, Professor Francis Pringle and Dr Francis Pringle.[5, 6]

Physician and Professor of Philosophy

On his return to Scotland in 1832 Pringle went into medical practice in Edinburgh.[7] He was involved in the third revision of the *Edinburgh Pharmacopoeia*, vowing to include 'only remedies with clear evidence of their worth,' so that many of the ancient remedies based on no more than tradition or superstition were removed. His background in philosophy facilitated his appointment as Professor of Ethics and Moral Philosophy in the University of Edinburgh, a post he held for eight years while continuing in practice as a physician.

Pringle moved in the circle of leading figures of the Scottish Enlightenment including David Hume, Adam Smith, William Cullen and the politician Andrew Mitchell.[8]

Physician General to the Army

In 1742, despite having no military experience or background, this philosopher/physician joined the British forces fighting the War of the Austrian Succession in Flanders. Pringle was appointed personal physician to Sir John Dalrymple (1673–1747) 2nd

4 M. A. Stewart, 'Berkeley and the Rankenian Club' in D. Berman (ed.), *George Berkeley, Essays and Replies* (Dublin: Irish Academic Press, 1986), pp.25–45.
5 Dorothea Waley Singer, 'Sir John Pringle and his circle. Part I, Life' in *Annals of Science*, 6:2 (1949), pp.127–180.
6 R. W. Innes Smith, *English Speaking Students of Medicine at the University of Leyden* (Edinburgh: Oliver and Boyd, 1932), p.187.
7 Kippis, *Six Discourses,* Preface, p.4.
8 Stewart, 'Berkeley and the Rankenian Club', pp.25–45.

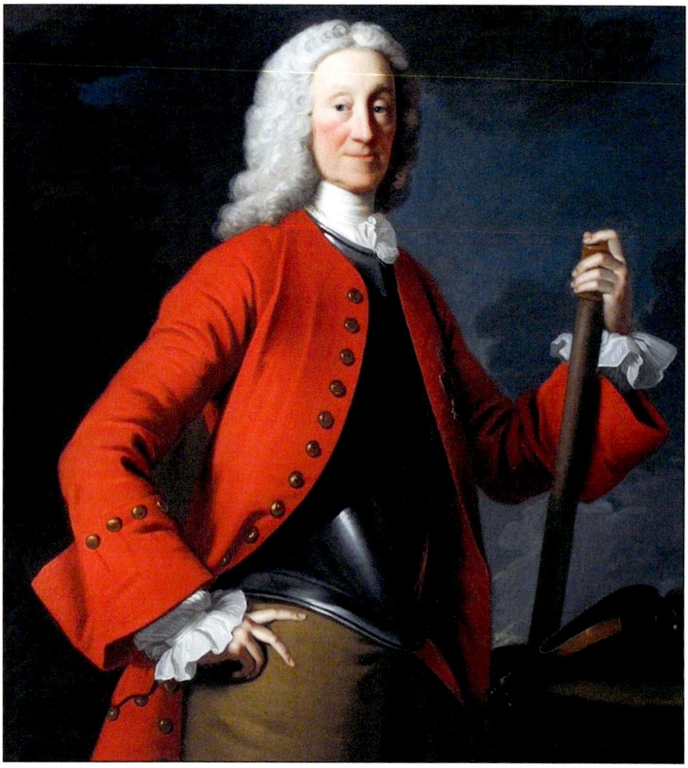

Field Marshal Sir John Dalrymple (1673–1747) 2nd Earl of Stair by Allan Ramsay. (National Trust for Scotland. Public Domain)

Earl of Stair, the Field Marshal commanding the British troops in Flanders. The Dalrymple and Pringle families were neighbours in the Scottish Borders and had been closely connected for generations.

This connection may have helped Pringle's subsequent appointment as Physician General to the Army in 1745, a post in which he had overall responsibility for all physicians in the army. Physicians were uncommon in the army as most medical care was carried out by regimental surgeons supported by surgeon's mates and orderlies. In his new role Pringle divided his time between Stair's military headquarters and the general hospital which had accompanied the army to Flanders, both of which were initially based in Ghent. General hospitals were generally located in large country houses or public buildings rented or commandeered for the purpose.[9] Pringle was keen to observe at first hand the medical conditions affecting the troops and arranged to share clinical duties with the hospital physician Dr Alexander Somerville.

9 Neil Cantlie, *A History of the Army Medical Department*, vol.1, (Edinburgh and London: Churchill Livingstone, 1974), p.89.

Observations on the Diseases of the Army

Pringle's observations on conditions affecting the soldiers began immediately. Most were detailed and astute and he recorded them assiduously. The importance of observation had been instilled into him from his studies of Bacon and of Sydenham and from the clinical teaching in Leiden.[10] His observations included not only symptoms and signs of illness but the context in which they occurred such as the timing, the location, the environment, the season and the meteorological conditions. In his recording, Pringle applied Baconian methodology to form hypotheses which he then tried to prove or disprove, and thereby draw conclusions which he hoped would help him in 'tracing causes of military distempers so as to suggest proper measures for preventing or lessening such causes in any future campaign.'[11]

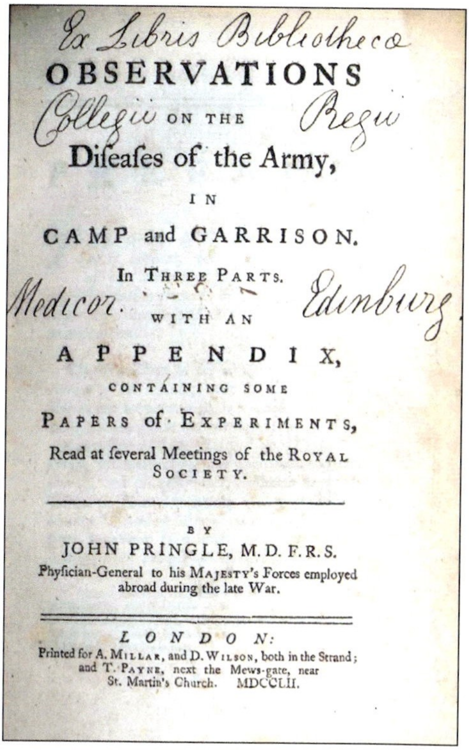
Ex Libris Bibliotheca Collegii Regii Medicor. Edinburg.

OBSERVATIONS

ON THE

Diseases of the Army,

IN

CAMP and GARRISON.

In THREE PARTS.

WITH AN

APPENDIX,

CONTAINING SOME

PAPERS of EXPERIMENTS,

Read at several Meetings of the ROYAL SOCIETY.

BY

JOHN PRINGLE, M. D. F. R. S.

Physician-General to his MAJESTY's Forces employed abroad during the late War.

LONDON:

Printed for A. MILLAR, and D. WILSON, both in the Strand; and T. PAYNE, next the Mews-gate, near St. Martin's Church. MDCCLII.

Frontispiece of *The Diseases of the Army in Camp and in Garrison*. 1st edition 1752.

It was Pringle's emphasis on finding the cause of disease that set him apart from most of his contemporaries. Only by finding the cause of a condition, he argued, could it be prevented.

In the preface of his magnum opus *Observations on the Diseases of the Army in Camp and in Garrison*, first published in 1752, he wrote 'There remains no account of the diseases incident to the armies of the ancients .... Nor has this deficiency been supplied .... by any of the moderns.'[12] This was essentially the first textbook of military medicine in the world. It is notable in many ways, not least because it includes descriptions of conditions such as fevers, fluxes and itch, outlining their clinical features, treatment, possible causes and prognosis. While such descriptions of disease are now the

10 For a fuller account of the influence of Sydenham on Pringle's thinking see Hilary Morris, *Military and Naval Campaigning on Behalf of the Health of Society, with Reference to Eighteenth and early Nineteenth Century Britain.* PhD thesis, University of Portsmouth. https://pure.port.ac.uk/ws/portalfiles/portal/11009512/ThesisPDF.pdf (accessed 23 November 2023).

11 John Pringle, *Observations on the Diseases of the Army*, 4th edition (London: Printed for A. Millar; D. Wilson, 1764), p.14.

12 Pringle, *Observations,* p.v.

norm in textbooks, in the mid-eighteen century this was an innovative, even radical, approach.

Pringle's book ran to seven English and three American editions and further editions in four major European languages. It was to prove hugely influential in Britain, Europe and America, not just during Pringle's lifetime but for decades afterwards. It stimulated further studies of military medicine such as those by the military physicians Richard Brocklesby (1722–1797), his successor as Physician General,[13] and by Donald Monro (1728–1802),[14] both published in 1764. The following year, in 1765, Pringle was acknowledged by the German physician Ernst Baldinger,[15] while in 1772 Jean Colombier, a French military physician, wrote that when 'Pringle gave his observations in 1752, all that had been done up until then seemed only a sketch too light to even consider.'[16] Pringle's influence is still evident in *Directions for Preserving the Health of Soldiers* written in 1778 by the prominent American physician Benjamin Rush (1748–1813), who had received his medical training in Edinburgh.[17]

While Pringle's observations included conditions like intermittent fevers (now believed to be malaria) and consumption (tuberculosis), this chapter will consider in detail three of the conditions he described, arguably the most common and most important; malignant fever (grouped with hospital, jail, camp, or ship fever), now thought to be epidemic typhus; flux, thought to be bacillary dysentery; and the itch now known to be scabies.

One of Pringle's first observations was that 'Hospitals are among the chief causes of sickness and death in the Army', and he set out to change that.[18]

Fevers

This was an age of classification but Pringle dismissed disease nosology writing, correctly as it turned out, 'diseases cannot be classified like plants.'

The term fever still gave rise to much confusion in the eighteenth century but Pringle was able to make some important groupings. Smallpox, measles and scarlet

13 Richard Brocklesby, *Oeconomical and Medical Observations, in Two Parts. From the Year 1758 to the Year 1763 Inclusive* (London: T. Becket & P.A De Hondt, 1764). http://hdl.handle.net/10713/1958 (accessed 23 November 2023)

14 Donald Monro, *Observations on the Means of Preserving the Health of Soldiers and of Conducting Military Hospitals,* (London: Murray, 1780).

15 Ernst Gottfried Baldinger, *Von den Krankheiten Einer Armee,* (Langensalza: Johann Christian Martini, 1774).

16 Jean Colombier, *Code de Médecine Militaire Pour le Service de Terre.* 5 tomes (Paris: J. P. Costard, 1772), vol. I, pp.x-xi.

17 Benjamin Rush, *Directions for Preserving the Health of Soldiers Recommended to the Consideration of the Officers of the Army of the United States,* (Lancaster, PA: Printed by John Dunlap, 1778) https://data.historicaltexts.jisc.ac.uk/view?pubId=eccoii-1377800200.

18 Pringle, *Observations,* p viii.

fever could readily be identified clinically and he recognised these as distinct entities. He recognised a further group of 'inflammatory fevers' where the condition appeared to affect one specific part of the body such as pneumonia or pleurisy. Most other fevers were thought to arise from noxious vapours, the 'miasma' which arose from stagnant marshes or other effluvia.

Within these fevers Pringle recognised two major groups. One included marsh fever, biliary fever, intermitting or remitting fever, so-called because of frequent relapses and this included the tertian or quartan forms, terms still in use today when describing the periodicity of febrile episodes in malaria. It is now believed that all that all of these terms were describing forms of malaria. Marsh fever was a recognition that the condition was often associated with damp, marshy environments while biliary fever was so-called because some patients became jaundiced, the result of haemolysis, the breaking down of red blood cells by malaria parasites.

Pringle observed that, 'If ever the fever appeared in a tertian or quartan form, after the usual evacuations the bark was a sure remedy,'[19] another reminder that Pringle, despite his empiricism, practised humoral medicine throughout his life. The 'usual evacuations' were bloodletting and purgation, but his observation – that the bark was a sure remedy for what we now know to be malaria – was an astute one. The bark was Jesuit or Cinchona bark whose active ingredient is now known to be quinine. Pringle's recommendation that it should be given in larger doses and for longer periods than was customary was probably responsible for his assertion that it was 'a sure remedy'.

He also recognised another important group of fevers encompassing malignant fever, hospital fever, jail fever, camp fever and ship fever, describing this as 'the most fatal distemper incident to the army.' Pringle's observations on this group led him to draw conclusions that were to advance our understanding of the causes and prevention of the infection now known as epidemic typhus.

Typhus, 'the most fatal distemper incident to the army'

Typhus in the Flanders Campaign

Pringle's first encounter with what he termed the 'malignant or hospital fever'[20] was at the general hospital in Ghent where many of those admitted with the condition died. After the Battle of Dettingen in June 1743, as the victorious army returned to its Flanders base, Pringle estimated that around half was afflicted with the fever. An unrecorded number died in regimental hospitals but of the estimated 5,000 admitted to local hospitals some 1,500 died, compared to 229 deaths on the battlefield.[21]

After the campaigning season ended Pringle introduced a number of reforms into the army medical services based on his observations. Having concluded that hospitals

19 Pringle, *Observations,* p.212.
20 Pringle, *Observations,* p.16.
21 McCrae, *Saving the Army,* p.73.

were the cause of much illness and specifically that overcrowding appeared to increase the incidence of malignant fever, he ordered that there must be greater spacing between individual soldiers in hospitals, camps and billets. He specified that each patient in a general hospital should have a minimum space of 36 square feet.[22] The effect of these and his other reforms were put to the test early in 1745 after the disastrous defeat at the Battle of Fontenoy, the bloodiest conflict of the campaign. It was estimated that the 20 British battalions had suffered over 4,000 killed or wounded. Yet in the aftermath of the battle there were no epidemics of fever and dysentery such as had been seen after Dettingen. Pringle was able to record that, 'By September few of the battalions had suffered more than twelve sick, a number as low as could be expected in the best of quarters.'[23] 'At the end of the campaign,' he noted with satisfaction that the three general hospitals had, 'about 1,000 sick, a small number when we consider that there had been in Flanders, beside the cavalry, 29 battalions'[24] – an estimated total of around 21,000 men. There had been a dramatic reduction in the incidence of disease since the epidemics that ravaged the army after Dettingen. Pringle recorded that, 'from the beginning to the end of the [Fontenoy] campaign, exclusive of those who were killed in battle or died of their wounds, the deaths did not exceed 200.'[25] A subsequent report by the Army Medical Board calculated that mortality of those admitted to general hospitals after Dettingen had been 21 percent whereas after the reforms it had fallen to 11 percent.[26] It was the first suggestion that these epidemic fevers could be prevented or at least significantly reduced by Pringle's reforms. These policies were soon to be put to further test, this time on the British mainland.

Typhus in the 1745–1746 Campaign to Suppress The Jacobite Rising

After the defeat of the Government Army of General Sir John Cope by the Jacobite army at Prestonpans in September 1745, the Government began to withdraw forces from Flanders to suppress the Jacobite rising (see map). Three battalions returned via Gravesend to Lichfield in the West Midlands where an army assembled under Sir John Ligonier. When the Duke of Cumberland returned from Flanders, he took command of this army and was joined by Pringle who stayed with him throughout the rest of the campaign. A further seven battalions returned to Berwick, Holy Island and Newcastle to join the army of Field Marshal Wade forming just outside Newcastle. The troops who arrived in Lichfield had had a brief journey across the Channel and were 'in perfect health'. Those heading for north-east England had set off in good health but had been delayed for several days by bad weather with the soldiers confined in overcrowded ships' holds. Those landing at Newcastle suffering from the 'malignant fever' were treated in a general hospital where the fever spread. Of the 96 soldiers with

22 McCrae, *Saving the Army,* p.80.
23 Pringle, *Observations,* p.36.
24 Pringle, *Observations,* p.74.
25 Pringle, *Observations,* p.74.
26 Cantlie, *History,* vol. 1, p.89.

the fever who landed at Holy Island, 40 died and the condition spread around the island, rapidly affecting one-sixth of its population. [27]

At Lichfield there was a later outbreak of continuous or 'jail-like' fever which filled the regimental hospitals and soon the poorhouse which served as a general hospital was also overcrowded. Pringle began to suspect that 'continuous', 'jail', and 'hospital fever' were all the same condition, characterised by high fever, headache, petechial rash, delirium and often death. Worse was to come. 'From the middle of February [1746]' Pringle wrote, 'when the army crossed the Forth, to the end of the campaign there had been in hospitals upwards of 2,000 men, including the wounded; of which number 300 died and mostly of this malignant fever.'[28]

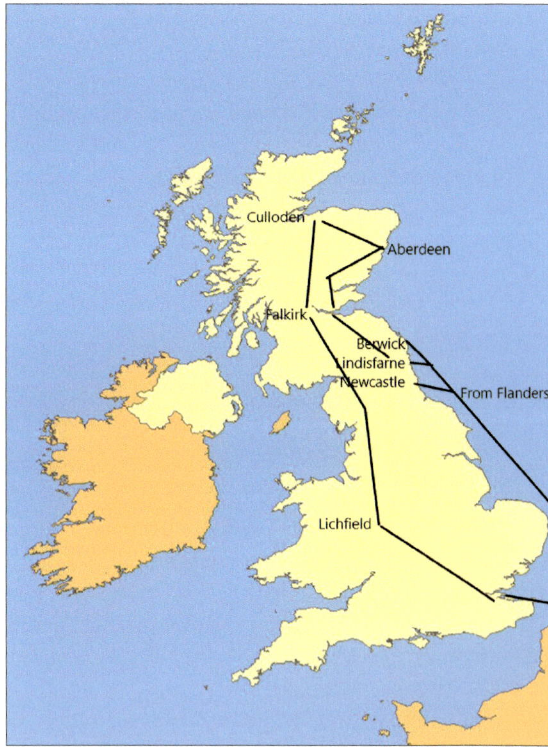

Government forces return from Flanders by several routes. Cumberland's army assembled at Lichfield in the West Midlands and Wade's outside Newcastle. (Author's diagram)

Having observed further outbreaks of ship, jail and camp fever he became convinced that all were the same condition. While caring for the sick at Nairn after the Battle of Culloden, he concluded that 'the symptoms of jail fever were in every point so like those of the hospital fever …that they were now proved to be really so.'[29] This was to be the first time this association had been established.

The Cause and Prevention of Malignant Fever

Pringle observed that these illnesses were associated with dirt, poor hygiene and overcrowding and concluded that this led to 'putrid air' which allowed the condition to spread. Yet he frequently used the phrase 'seeds of disease' which he believed carried disease from person to person.

27 Pringle, Observations, p.40.
28 Pringle, *Observations,* p.53.
29 Pringle, *Observations,* p.48.

Later, in a letter to Richard Mead in 1750, he set out detailed recommendations for the prevention of the condition:

> Allow no prisoner to carry out his cloaths; which should be burnt, and supplied by others, at the publick expense; secondly, to order, that the cloaths of malefactors, after execution, should be also burnt; but above all, that before prisoners are brought into the court, they should be cleaned and put in cloaths to be kept for that purpose, and washed from time to time.[30]

The measures which Pringle recommended should have reduced the spread of typhus, yet it continued to plague armies until the First World War, despite the revelation in the early years of the twentieth century that it was a bacterial infection whose main vector was the body louse.

The flux

An epidemic of 'bloody dysentery' in the days after the victory at Dettingen was Pringle's first encounter with 'flux' in the army. Although germ theory would not become established for over a century, Pringle came very close to an understanding of the way that it spread:

> In camp the **contagion** passes from one who is ill to his companions in the same tent and from thence to the next. The foul straw becomes very **infectious**. But the great **source of infection** are the privvies after they have received the excrement of those who first fall ill.[31] [Author's emphases]

As a result of these observations, he was able to order preventive measures – that bedding straw should be frequently changed, that the latrine pits should be dug far from camp and earthed over each day and that there should be greater spacing in camps, hospitals and billets. A further preventative measure was well ahead of its time:

> The faeces are rendered less, if at all infectious, by means of a strong acid combined with the parts that are really septic – especially, in the dysentery, where the faeces are highly corrupted and contagious.[32]

30 John Pringle, *On the Nature and Cure of Hospital and Jayl-Fevers. Letter to Doctor Mead.* (London: A Miller & D Wilson, 1750), p.50.
31 Pringle, *Observations,* pp.263–264.
32 Pringle, *Observations,* p.103.

It seems that Joseph Lister, a century later, was unaware of this innovation when he wrote 'I was much struck with an account of the remarkable effects produced by carbolic acid upon the sewage [in Carlisle],' an observation which would eventually lead to antiseptic surgery.[33]

Pringle considered possible causes of dysentery and concluded that he was, 'in favour of Kircher's system of contagion by animalcules.' Athanasius Kircher (1602–1680), a Jesuit scholar who had examined the blood of plague victims under the microscope, described 'little worms which propagate plague', one of the first expressions of the concept of germ theory.[34]

Yet despite the reforms Pringle introduced to reduce the incidence of dysentery, the army continued to experience epidemics well into the next century, probably because the importance of hand washing was not appreciated.

The itch

Pringle's observations of the itch, now known to be scabies, led him close to a true understanding of its aetiology. There was an outbreak of the itch as soon as British troops began to arrive in Flanders in the summer of 1742 and this continued throughout the campaign. Pringle observed that this was, 'the most general distemper among soldiers.' He appreciated that the spread was person to person, recording that it was due to the 'contagion of a few who having the distemper before the embarkation communicated it to their companions on board the ships and in the barracks after their arrival.'[35]

He made a further important observation:

> Although it be of a **contagious** nature, the infection is communicated only by the **contact** of the diseased person, of his clothes bedding et cetera and **not by effluvia** as in the dysentery and malignant fever.[36] [Author's emphasis]

He concluded from this that the condition, 'seems best accounted for by Leeuwenhoek from certain small insects he discovered in the pustules by the microscope.'[37] Antonie van Leeuwenhoek (1632–1723) a Dutch merchant had developed an early microscope and used this to study human and plant tissues, making drawings of his findings. Some of the drawings which Leeuwenhoek made of organisms in the pus from scabies

33 Joseph Lister, 'On a New Method of Treating Compound Fracture, Abscess, etc.' *The Lancet*. I (London: 1867), pp.326, 357, 387, 507.
34 Athanasius Kircher, *Scrutinium Physicio-Medicum Contagiosae Luis, Quae Pestis Dicitur*, (Rome: Mascardi, 1658).
35 Pringle, *Observations*, p.15.
36 Pringle, *Observations*, p.350.
37 Pringle, *Observations*, p.350.

sores bear a very close resemblance to the scabies mite.[38] Pringle was also aware of the description and drawings made in 1681 by Bonomo[39] and Cestoni of 'very minute living creatures' which had been isolated from scabies pustules and viewed under an early microscope.[40] Bonomo's original letter had been translated by Pringle's friend Richard Mead.[41]

Pringle's views on the treatment of scabies were clear. Sulphur was the specific remedy being, 'more safe and more efficacious than mercury,' although he realised that sometimes, 'the animalcula may lie too deep to be destroyed by an external application.'[42] His conviction that sulphur was the specific treatment and was safer and more effective than mercury was ahead of its time. An article published in 2022 in a specialist dermatology journal showed a 10 percent sulphur ointment was significantly more effective in treating scabies than 5 percent permethrin cream, the NICE recommended first line treatment. The authors conclude that 10 percent sulphur ointment, 'can be considered a safe and effective topical option in the treatment of scabies' – conclusions strikingly similar to Pringle's some 275 years earlier![43]

Pringle made other reforms. His proposal during the Dettingen campaign that military hospitals should be neutral, exempted from attack and should treat enemy wounded was a radical one based on his humanitarian ideals. It was respected during the campaign but fell into abeyance until the first Geneva Convention – 120 years later! His ideals also led to reforms in the general health, hygiene and welfare of the troops such as improving their diet, ensuring that they had greater protection from cold and wet and that on return to camp they cleaned in warm water and had fresh linen.

Later career

After his army service Pringle became a physician in London, eventually becoming physician to King George III. His enquiring mind continued to pursue the causes and

38 Antoni van Leeuwenhoek, 'An Abstract of a Letter from Mr Anthony von Leevvenhoeck at Delft, dated Sep. 17. 1683' in *Philosophical Transactions of the Royal Society of London.* 14 (London: 1684) pp.568–574.

39 Pringle, *Observations,* p.350.

40 M. A. Montesu, F. Cottoni, 'G. C. Bonomo and D. Cestoni. Discoverers of the Parasitic Origin of Scabies' in *American. Journal of Dermatopathology,* 13 (Philadelphia: 1991), pp.425–427.

41 Richard Mead, 'An Abstract of Part of a Letter from Dr Bonomo to Signior Redi, containing some observations concerning the worms of humane bodies' in *Philosophical Transactions of the. Royal Society* 23 (London: 1703) pp.1296–1299. http://doi.org/10.1098/rstl.1702.0040 (accessed 21 December 2023).

42 Pringle, *Observations,* p.353.

43 G. Ertugrul & H. Aktas, 'Comparison of Sulfur Ointment and Permethrin Treatments in Scabies' in *Dermatology Therapy,* 35; 12 (Newark NJ: 2022). https://pubmed.ncbi.nlm.nih.gov/36193643 (accessed 23 December 2023).

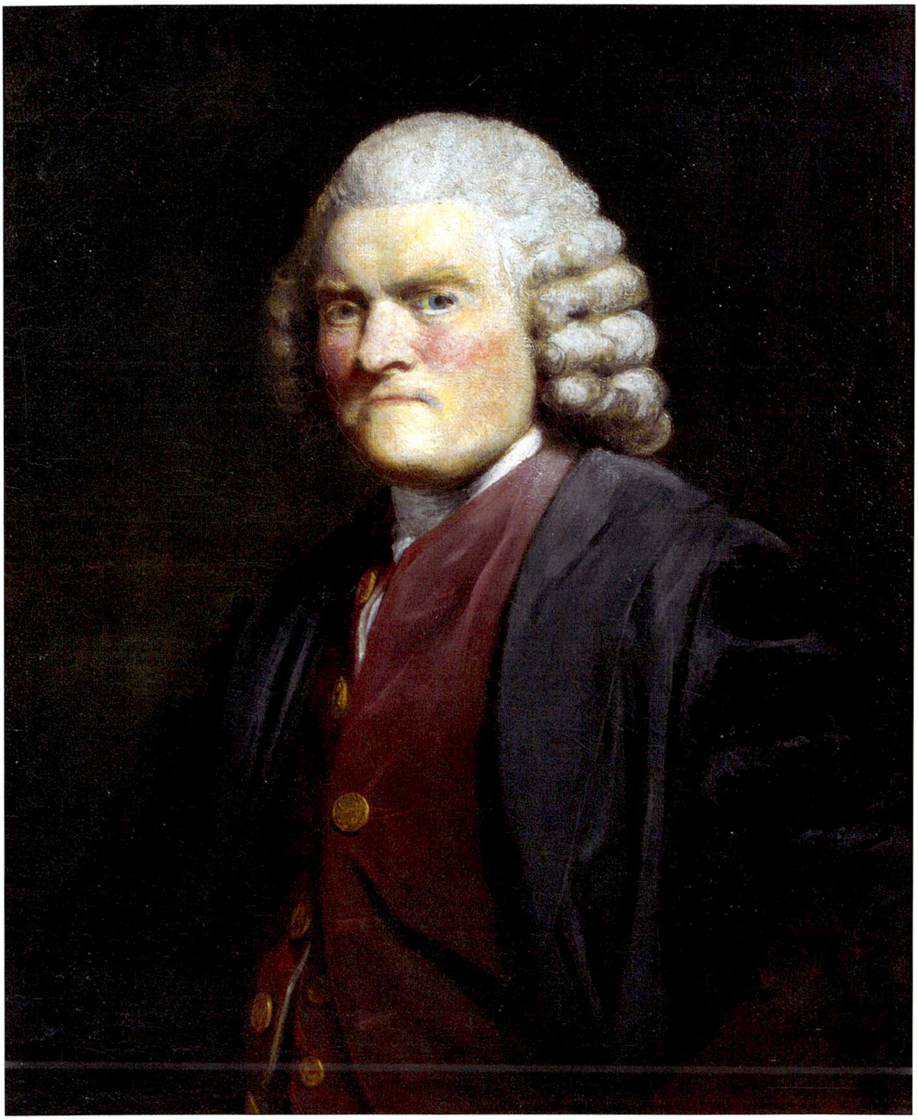

Sir John Pringle in later life, by Joshua Reynolds.
(With kind permission of The Royal Society)

prevention of putrefaction in a series of elegant laboratory experiments. He compared the efficacy of acids and alkalis in preventing putrefaction, coining the terms 'septic' and 'antiseptic' to describe these[44] and concluding that among the most potent antiseptics were borax and alum. For this and other experimental work he was awarded the prestigious Copley Medal by the Royal Society in 1752.

Conclusion

Pringle developed and promoted Baconian thinking in medicine, was influential in the epistemological change that took place in medicine in the eighteenth century, largely due to the impact of his book *Observations,* effectively the first textbook of military medicine. Notably he was able to use reason and logic to introduce hygiene reforms, firstly in the army and later in civilian practice, as measures to prevent communicable disease. His contributions to the prevention of disease in military medicine were arguably the greatest made in the eighteenth century.

Bibliography

Books

Baldinger, E. G., *Von den Krankheiten Einer Armee* (Langensalza; Martini, 1774)

Brocklesby, Richard, *Oeconomical and Medical Observations, in Two Parts. From the Year 1758 to the Year 1763 Inclusive* (London: Becket & de Hondt, 1764)

Cantlie, Neil, *A History of the Army Medical Department* (Edinburgh and London: Churchill Livingstone, 1974) 2 volumes

Colombier, Jean, *Code de Médecine Militaire Pour le Service de Terre,* 5 tomes, (Paris, J.-P. Costard, 1772), vol. I pp.x–xi

Innes Smith, R. W., *English Speaking Students of Medicine at the University of Leyden* (Edinburgh: Oliver and Boyd, 1932)

Kippis, Andrew, *Six Discourses delivered by Sir John Pringle, Bart* (London: W. Strahan and T. Cadell, 1783)

Kircher, Athanasius, *Scrutinium Physicio-Medicum Contagiosae Luis, Quae Pestis Dicitur* (Rome: Mascardi, 1658)

McCrae, Morrice, *Saving the Army: The Life of Sir John Pringle* (Edinburgh: John Donald, 2014)

Monro, Donald, *Observations on the Means of Preserving the Health of Soldiers and of Conducting Military Hospitals* (London: Murray, 1780)

Pringle, John, *Observations on the Diseases of the Army, in Camp and Garrison. In Three Parts* (London: Millar, Wilson & Payne, 1752)

44 Pringle, *Observations,* p.482.

Pringle, John, *On the Nature and Cure of Hospital and Jayl-Fevers. Letter to Doctor Mead* (London: A Miller & D Wilson, 1750)

Rush, Benjamin, *Directions for Preserving the Health of Soldiers Recommended to the Consideration of the Officers of the Army of the United States,* (Lancaster, PA: printed by John Dunlap, 1778) https://data.historicaltexts.jisc.ac.uk/view?pubId=eccoii-1377800200

Book chapters

Stewart, M. A., 'Berkeley and the Rankenian Club' in D. Berman (ed.), *George Berkeley, Essays and Replies* (Dublin: Irish Academic Press, 1986), pp.25–45

Journal articles

Ertugrul G & Aktas H., 'Comparison of Sulfur Ointment and Permethrin Treatments in Scabies' in *Dermatology Therapy*, 35:12 (Newark, NJ: 2022), https://pubmed.ncbi.nlm.nih.gov/36193643/ (accessed 23 December 2023)

van Leeuwenhoek, Antoni, 'An abstract of a letter from Mr. Anthony von Leevvenhoeck at Delft, dated Sep. 17. 1683' in *Philosophical Transactions of the Royal Society of London,* 14 (London: 1684), pp.568–574

Lister, J., 'On a new method of treating compound fracture, abscess, etc.' in *The Lancet*, 1 (London: 1867), pp.326, 357, 387, 507

Macintyre, Iain, 'A sceptic and an Empiric in Medicine: George Young (1692–1757) and the Beginnings of the Scottish medical Enlightenment' in *Journal of the Royal College of Physicians of Edinburgh,* 42: 4 (Edinburgh: 2012), pp.352–60

Mead, Richard, 'An Abstract of Part of a Letter from Dr Bonomo to Signior Redi, Containing Some Observations Concerning the Worms of Humane Bodies' in *Philosophical Transactions of the Royal Society,* 23 (London: 1703) pp.1296–1299 http://doi.org/10.1098/rstl.1702.0040 (accessed 21 December 2023)

Montesu, M. A., Cottoni, F., 'G. C. Bonomo and D. Cestoni. Discoverers of the parasitic origin of scabies' in *American Journal of Dermatopathology,* 13 (Philadelphia: 1991), pp.425–427

Singer, Dorothea W., 'Sir John Pringle and His Circle. Part I, Life,' in *Annals of Science*, 6:2 (1949), pp.127–180

Dissertations

Morris, Hilary, 'Military and Naval Campaigning on Behalf of the Health of Society, with reference to eighteenth and early nineteenth century Britain.' PhD thesis, University of Portsmouth https://pure.port.ac.uk/ws/portalfiles/portal/11009512/ThesisPDF.pdf. (accessed 23 November 2023)

2

Legacy and Learning: Military Surgical Practice 1756–1815

Mick Crumplin

Before the advent of anaesthesia and antiseptic surgical practice, military surgical advances were limited. Understanding of the pathophysiology of combat trauma evolved over the twentieth century and continues to do so. However, during the eighteenth and early nineteenth centuries when large numbers of battle casualties were sustained, there were some isolated improvements based on empiricism and reasoning that would benefit both surgeons and their charges. For three centuries, Scotland's contributions to medicine and surgery were disproportionally high in Britain. For example, during the final year of the Napoleonic War, while Scotland's populace was only 11 percent of that of Great Britain, 40 percent of surgeons (103 out of 255) serving in Wellington's Allied Army during the Waterloo campaign (15 June to 8 July 1815) were either Scots or had received their essential surgical training and qualification north of the border.[1] The prominent roles of the parish school system and the dominie, a high literacy rate and a generous provision of universities ensured a significant presence of Scots professionals worldwide.

Surgical Education and Training

What contributions then were made to military surgical practice by Scots surgeons? Before and after qualification, a sound knowledge of anatomy for any operative procedure was, and still is, integral to surgical operations. Physiology and pathology were as yet rudimentary. Teaching of anatomy and surgery was performed by cadaveric dissection, assisted by the use of texts, illustrative works and wax or wooden models. On the battlefield, much accrued field experience replaced limited learning of operative surgery in the civilian setting. On campaign, for the junior surgeons assisting

1 M. K. H. Crumplin, *The Bloody Fields of Waterloo, Medical Support for Wellington's Greatest Battle* (Huntingdon: Ken Trotman Publishing, 2015), data from pp.148–240.

seniors was invaluable experience. Post mortem dissections and reports on the 'education abilities' of medical officers had been encouraged by Sir James McGrigor (1771–1815) in the Peninsular War of 1808–1814.[2] Burgeoning use of statistics occurred towards the end of those campaigns. For the most part we rely on the more successful and prominent military surgeons' publications and case notes, so unfortunately the surgical performance of many 'ordinary' serving regimental and staff surgeons remains unavailable.

Some Scottish Contributors to Military Surgery

The following discussion therefore highlights the contributions and some aspects of practice of some of the major contributors to surgical education and practice, providing reference to their particular works, as appropriate. This includes the Hunter brothers, particularly John Hunter (1728–1793), Benjamin Bell (1749–1806), John Bell (1763–1820), Sir James Wylie (1768–1854), George Guthrie (1785–1856) and will also touch on surgical benefits emanating from some of the men covered by the other contributors, where relevant. John Hennen (1779–1828) is also worthy of mention as, although Irish-born, it was in Edinburgh that he qualified, received his MD, was elected FRSE and taught military surgery. He wrote an invaluable and seminal work on military surgery.

Sir John Pringle (1707–1782) as a very able physician, proposed sanctuary and protection for field hospitals and the wounded, also he researched and worked on infection (particularly typhus) and made some valuable measures to preserve the army's health – issues covering hospital care, diet and hygiene were all beneficial to surgical cases.

William and John Hunter

The Hunter brothers, William (1718–1783) and John were raised in Long Calderwood, near the present-day East Kilbride. William was the first to emigrate to England and before long, evolving appropriate mannerisms and social skills, he proved an able man-midwife, physician and anatomist. Most importantly, he established a school of anatomy at Covent Garden then later, moving to Soho, he founded the Great Windmill School.

John, 10 years younger than his brother and an apprentice carpenter, joined William to assist with the running and work of the school. Less elegant than his brother and retaining his Scots accent, he soon became adept at specimen procurement and

2 J. McGrigor, *Instructions for the Regulation of Military Hospitals and the Sick with Divisions of the Army in the Peninsula* (Lisbon: printed by Antonio Rodrigues Galhardo, 1813), pp.19 & 26.

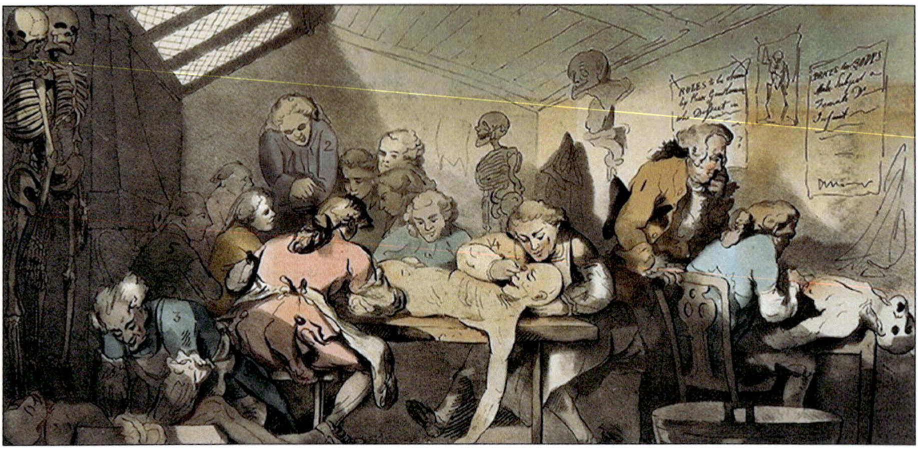

William Hunter, standing on left and John immediately to his left. Both brothers teaching while dissecting at their anatomy school. Aquatint by T. Rowlandson. (Author's collection)

preparation. John showed great interest and enquiry in animal and human anatomy and œconomy. His keen sense of observation and scientific reasoning were to bring him to prominence. The brothers' anatomy schools in London with their dissecting rooms, taught and influenced many aspiring military and civilian surgeons.[3]

John, eager to pursue a surgical career, was taught by such influential surgeons as Percival Pott (1714–1788) and William Cheselden (1688–1752) and took on a junior surgical position at St George's Hospital. There were few capital (major) operations to be witnessed in civilian practice, although John would have experienced some at the sides of Pott and Cheselden.

However, after more than a decade at the Covent Garden School, John was keen to further expand his surgical experience and joined the army as a hospital surgeon in 1761, during the Seven Years War (1756–1763). In 1761, he joined the combined operation expedition to capture Belle-Île, off the coast of Brittany. After a failed landing on the south of the island, the citadel and capital at Palais fell to General Studholme Hodgson (1708–1798). John became distressed at the rather meddlesome and rough surgery he witnessed. He decried the unnecessary and early interventions and became rather unpopular with some of his colleagues for his incisive views.[4]

With the relatively low energy transfer of muzzle-loading flintlock muskets, many wounds were caused by 'spent' rounds and men would have survived such wounds with conservative management. The medical staff on the island had around 500 casualties to treat shared between about 25 regimental and staff surgeons, thus the workload was not onerous and Hunter's experience was limited. One important oversight in his surgical practice was that, while he did categorise a few cases that would benefit from

3 Wendy Moore, *The Knife Man* (London: Bantam Press, 2005), p.40.
4 Moore, *The Knife Man*, pp.131–136.

John Hunter. (Collection of the Royal College of Surgeons of England, reproduced with permission)

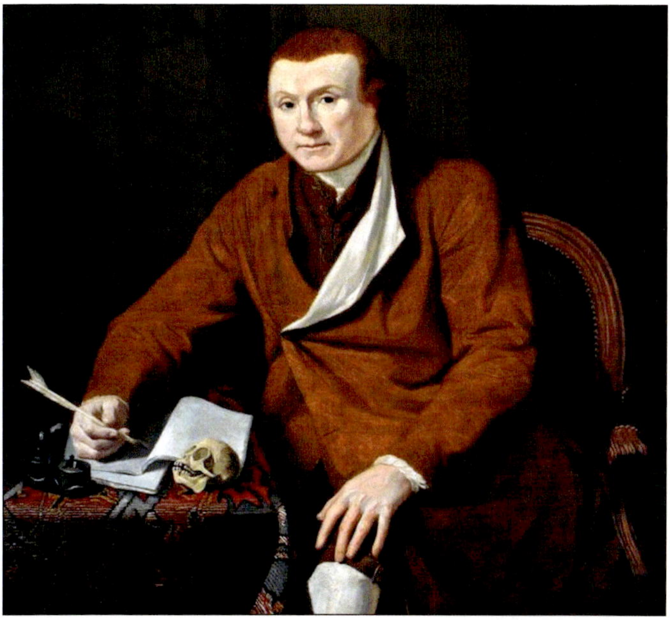

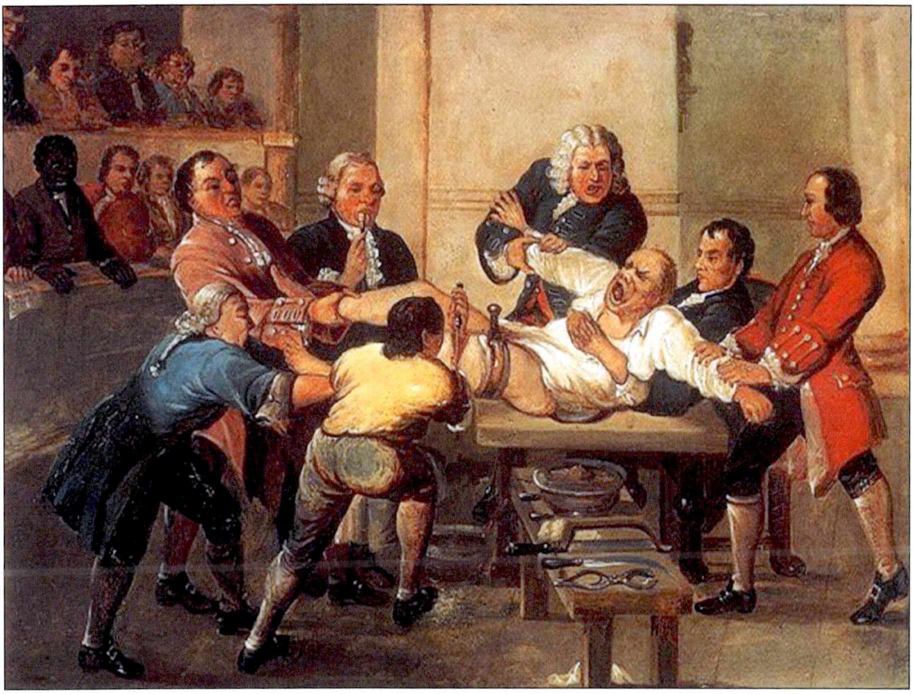

A mid-eighteenth century amputation. Painting, oil on wood, anonymous. (Collection of the Royal College of Surgeons of England, reproduced with permission)

early amputation, he mistakenly counselled that surgery should be delayed until after inflammatory changes had resolved.[5] He also laid down criteria for wound exploration warning of unnecessary surgical intervention.[6] Although promoting venesection, he cautioned against its use in certain cases.[7] Overall, we see a surgeon imbued with intelligence and reasoning, ready to challenge any blind illogical surgical dogma – the very essence of an Enlightenment surgeon.

John Hunter, by dint of his later established surgical reputation and military experiences, was promoted Surgeon General to the Army in 1790, but died three years later. He left important legacies for the proper governance and training of surgeons in the Army Medical Department. For example, he ensured that promotions and appointments should be solely carried out by the Army Medical Board, and junior surgeons should, as they do today at an early stage, experience time in a general hospital. Hunter believed that the best technical surgeons should work in larger hospitals and importantly, he saw promotion being earned by merit, not merely by seniority or patronage.[8]

Improving Surgical Care

As surgeons were often challenged by large numbers of casualties on the field, it is useful to consider what improvements in medical care could have been achieved at the time. Improvements could have included more precise indications for and the proper timing of amputations; retaining a limb or parts of it where feasible; better immobilisation of fractures; removing septic material indriven by missiles; developing clearer indications for trephining; caution with the liberal use of venesection; recording surgical data and, importantly, treating casualties where feasible, as close to the fighting as possible. Certainly the need to return men to the front as soon as it was possible, would boost a fighting force and this always remains an important military medical paradigm.

Three Surgical Bells

Although not directly affiliated with the army, Benjamin Bell (1749–1806) was considered a leading Edinburgh scientific surgeon. He promoted the saving of skin and soft tissue in surgery, perioperative pain relief and demonstrated that syphilis and gonorrhoea were different diseases. His seven-volume *System of Surgery* extended

5 E. Home, *A Treatise on the Blood, Inflammation and Gunshot Wounds*, by the Late John Hunter (London: printed by John Richardson, 1794), pp.560–563.
6 Home, *A Treatise*, pp.534–537.
7 Home, *A Treatise*, pp.563–564.
8 N. Cantlie, *A History of the Army Medical Department* (London and Edinburgh: Churchill Livingstone, 1974), vol. 1, p.171.

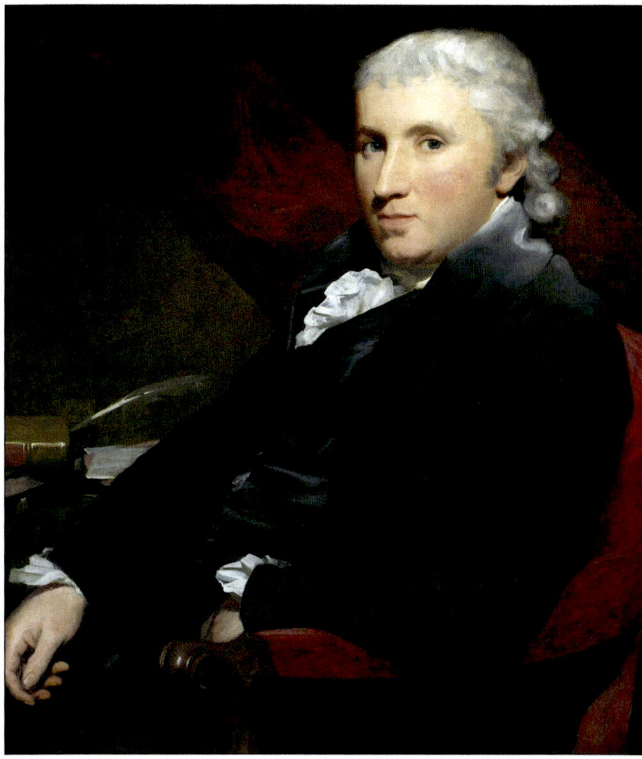

Benjamin Bell, oil painting by Allan Ramsay. (Professor James Garden, reproduced with permission)

to seven British editions, three American editions and was translated into Italian, French, Spanish, German, and it remained a recommended and popular text for military surgeons. The volumes covered regional injuries, gunshot wounds, burns and operative surgical procedures and all but two of the volumes were carefully illustrated.

John Bell (1763–1820) was not related to Benjamin but was the older brother of the talented artist, researcher, anatomist and surgeon, Sir Charles Bell. John Bell was a prominent and very talented and popular Edinburgh anatomist and surgeon, who opposed the University Professor of Medicine James Gregory (1753–1821) over staffing issues in the Edinburgh Royal Infirmary.[9]

John lectured and wrote in particular upon surgical anatomy and worked in his extramural school for around 13 years. Less well known as a draughtsman than Charles, his artistic talents were considerable.

His influential *Textbook of Surgery* also remained essential reading material for many an aspirant military doctor. It included views on vascular injuries and battlefield trauma. Perhaps one of the most important contributions John made to military medicine was

9 M.H. Kaufman, *The Regius Chair of Military Surgery in the University of Edinburgh 1806–1855* (Amsterdam & New York: Rodopi B.V, 2003), p.56.

a memorial written to the then First Lord of the Admiralty, Lord Spencer, in 1798 following the naval Battle of Camperdown in 1797 and John's observations on the management of the casualties in Yarmouth. He pleaded for a better system of military medical instruction.[10] This was a catalyst for the establishment of a Chair of Military Surgery later to be founded at the University of Edinburgh in 1806 (see Chapter 8).

Charles Bell, who was apprenticed to John, became a brilliant, talented and charismatic teacher and surgeon – his career is detailed in Chapter 7. He took over the Windmill Anatomy School and co-founded the Middlesex Hospital Medical School.

Relevant to his surgical contributions, were his lectures, writings and importantly his beautifully presented sketches, and paintings in both oils and watercolours.[11] These series were used as teaching aids and were made following visits to Portsmouth and Brussels, after the retreat from Corunna in 1809 and the Waterloo campaign in 1815 respectively.

He created generously illustrated texts, but especially useful to trainee surgeons were those in the *Great Operations of Surgery*,[12] which are still informative to modern medical historians.

Somewhat critical at times of contemporary military surgical practice, he lacked experience in that specialist field. Later in his remarkable career as a surgeon, artist and physiologist, he served as the first Professor of Surgery and Anatomy at the London College of Surgeons and then had a Chair in Surgery at the University of Edinburgh.

The Regius Chair of Military Surgery at Edinburgh University

A significant contribution to surgical tuition evolved from the Regius Chair of Military Surgery, which ran from 1806 to 1855, thus covering the last nine years of the Napoleonic Wars. This is described in detail in Chapter 8, but suffice it to say the teaching delivered at this institution influenced many young military doctors. Prior to the arrival of the Regius Chair, many military men throughout the nation complained of the absence of such an establishment in England, and the Chair further stimulated the migration of a large number of surgical trainees north of the border. The Chair was held by two men, Professor John Thomson (1765–1836), who held the position for 19 years until Sir George Ballingall (1780–1855) succeeded him. The Chair was abolished after the Crimean War upon Ballingall's death.[13]

10 Kaufman, *The Regius Chair*, pp.50–51.

11 T. Longmore, *Description of a Series of Watercolour Drawings Executed by the Late Sir Charles Bell, Illustrative of Wounds Received at the Battle of Waterloo* (Army Medical School Museum: 1816, cited in the Army Medical Department Report), Vol. VII, p.596.

12 C. Bell, *Illustrations of the Great Operations of Surgery* (London: Longman, Hurst, Rees Orme and Brown, 1821).

13 Kaufman, *The Regius Chair*, pp.189–193.

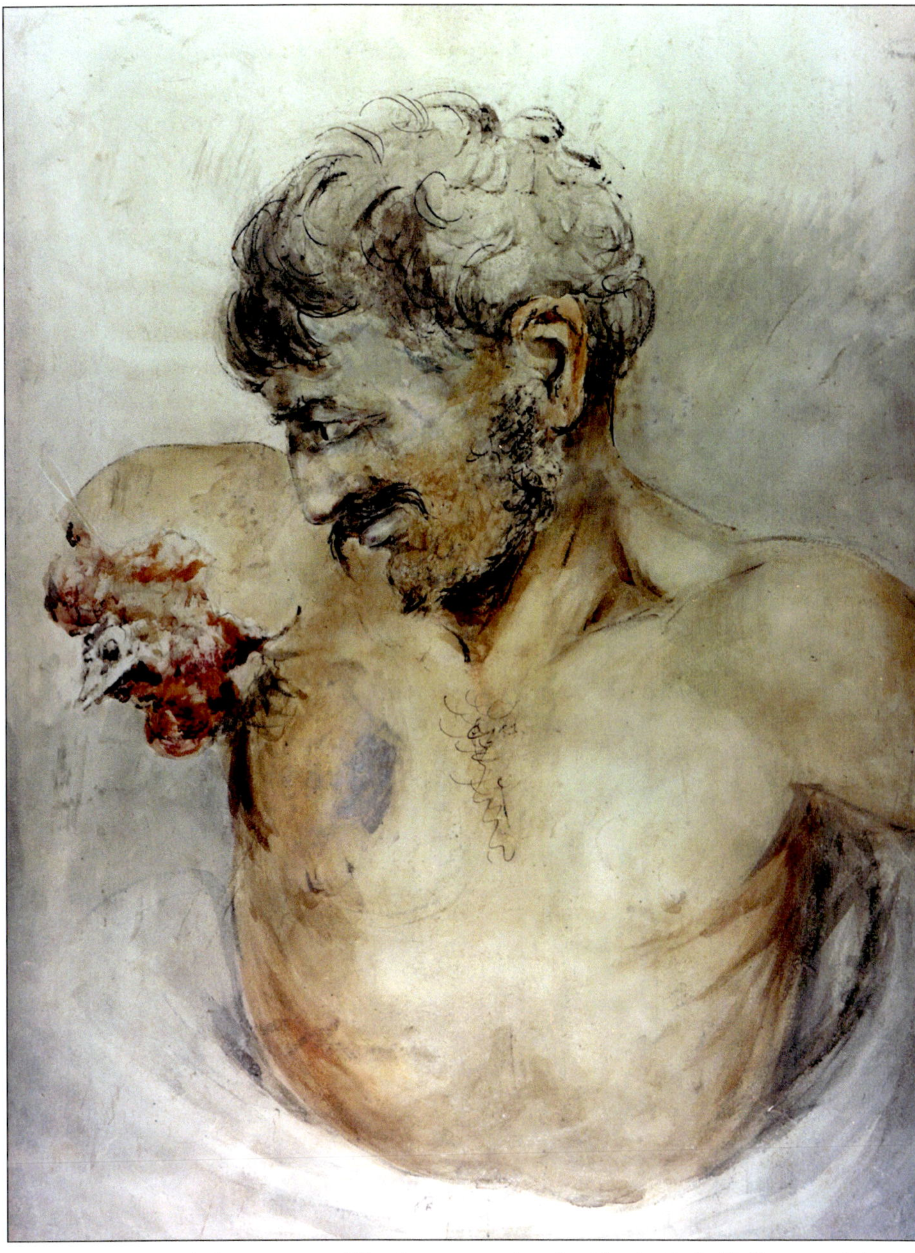

Hussar – round shot injury at Waterloo, watercolour by Charles Bell. (Collection of the Museum of Military Medicine, reproduced with permission)

Sir James Wylie

It is no understatement to say that Scots professional men influenced development of surgery on an international basis and the career of Sir James Wylie (1768–1854) is a notable example. He studied medicine in Edinburgh and qualified from the University of Aberdeen. Wylie was invited to work in Russia by the Scottish doctor John Rogerson, who was serving as a Physician to Catherine the Great (r.1762–1796) at the Imperial Court. He accepted the invitation and was later made senior surgeon to a Russian line regiment. Here he was soon recognised as an effective military physician and surgeon and received promotions. He served as medical officer to the Russian Imperial Guard and was present at the Battles of Austerlitz and Borodino. An effective teacher, he researched and published works on contagious diseases and field surgery. In 1823, he created the *Journal of Military Medicine*, still published today, the oldest Russian military medical journal. He held the post of President of the Russian Imperial Medical and Surgical Academy for 30 years (1808–1838).

George James Guthrie

There remains little doubt that George James Guthrie (1785–1856) was the ablest British military surgeon during the eighteenth century. Descended from an old Forfar family, and born in London of Scottish parents, Guthrie had a sound education from a French émigré. He went on to be the youngest surgeon to qualify at the London College of Surgeons at just under 16 years old. Serving at first as a regimental surgeon, he served through the Peninsular campaigns of 1808 to 1814, gaining a prodigious amount of experience. He expanded his burgeoning practice by operating upon and managing thousands of wounded and sick soldiers as a staff surgeon. Rather like John Hunter and John Bell, Guthrie could be highly critical of his surgical colleagues. Nevertheless, he proved to be a man of considerable skill and integrity and was also proficient in several languages.

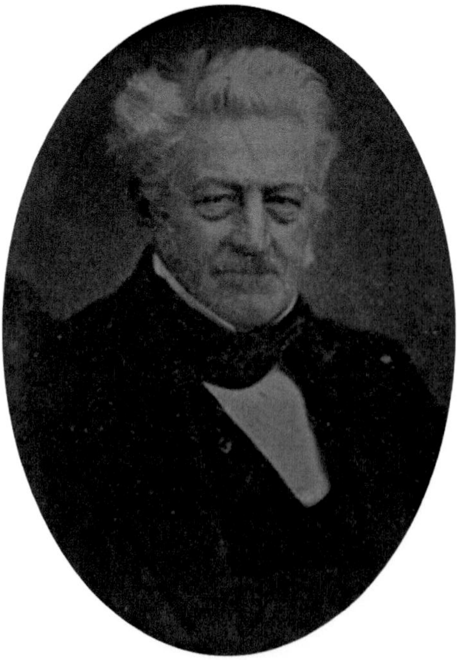

George James Guthrie at the age of 66, Daguerreotype. (Collection of the Royal College of Surgeons of England, reproduced with permission)

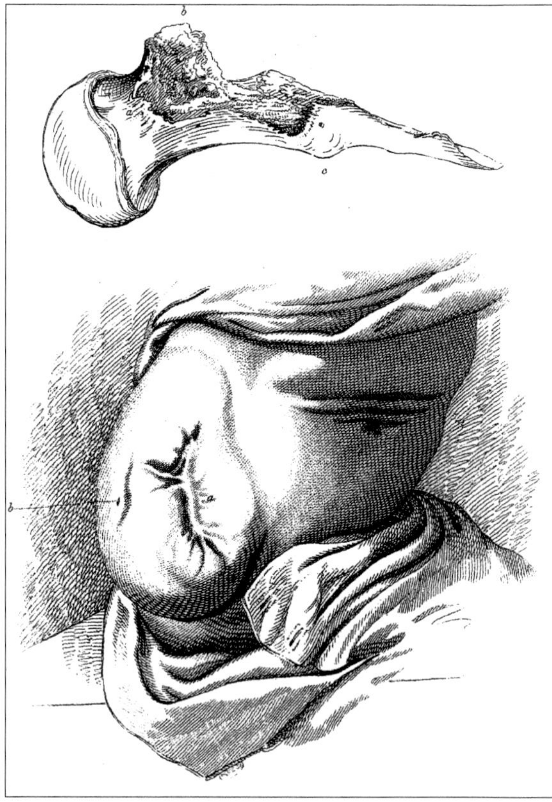

The scar and excised bone following disarticulation at the hip-joint by Guthrie. (Courtesy of Professor M. H. Kaufman)

His contributions to military surgical practice included clarifying indications for surgical intervention; operating as soon as the patient was reasonably stable after injury; conserving only useful limbs; controlling bleeding when operating without a tourniquet also ligating a blood vessel at either side of an injury.

He promoted the use of long limb splints, which although not ideal, were an improvement on the short military splints. In 1812, he performed and recorded a fasciotomy (soft tissue release) on a limb threatened by ischaemia caused by the skin infection erysipelas. He took a particular interest in chest injuries and in 1815, after Waterloo, he carried out the first successfully recorded surgical disarticulation at the hip-joint.

Other contributions to military surgery were his compilation of surgical outcomes at field and hospital operations and mortality figures. He studied post mortem material and carried out a simple trial of surgical and conservative therapy in the management of compound femoral fractures. Gaining further promotion, he left the army and, following the Battle of Waterloo, he became a surgeon at the Westminster Hospital.[14]

Guthrie continued to teach aspiring military men after the war using his extensive experience and a plethora of case reports. His lectures at the London College of Surgeons were given *gratis* to those serving in the armed forces or in the East India Company. The lectures, given from 1816 to the 1830s, were always well attended, not only for their high quality but also because Guthrie, being a somewhat robust (but fair) examiner, was not allowed to examine candidates who had attended his lectures.

14 M. Crumplin, *Guthrie's War, a Surgeon of the Peninsula and Waterloo* (Barnsley: Pen & Sword Books Ltd, 2010), p.160.

Guthrie's extensive list of publications included his book *Commentaries on the Surgery of the War*, which was published in six editions and was used well into the nineteenth century.[15] As to his later surgical career he helped found the Westminster Eye Hospital, was closely involved in the 1832 Anatomy Act, became the President of the London (later the English) College of Surgeons three times and took a special interest in ophthalmic surgery. This latter specialist commitment might seem unusual for a robust military surgeon, but might have been apposite since, after the Battle of Talavera in 1809, a witness observed Guthrie, who had just performed a trepanation of his patient, gently brushing away a blood clot from the surface of the man's brain using a feather!

Conclusion

In summary there were pivotal Scots figures who contributed to military surgical practice before the introduction of anaesthesia and antiseptic practice. Teaching basic surgical sciences, most particularly anatomy, were the Hunter and the Bell brothers and also John Thomson. As to military surgical teaching there were the experiences of Guthrie, Hennen, Thomson, Charles Bell, and James Wylie. The Bell brothers, Benjamin Bell and Thomson either proved themselves able draughtsmen or made wax models for teaching purposes. Both John Hunter and Sir James McGrigor introduced governance and regulation to military medicine and surgical practice and finally, John Hunter, McGrigor, Guthrie, Thomson, Hennen and Wylie all left their marks as experienced serving medical field officers.

In conclusion there is little doubt that through its sound educational system and a nation keen to provide competent professionals, Scotland at these times had contributed more than its fair share to support military medicine and would continue to do so in later years.

Bibliography

Primary Sources

Bell, C., *Illustrations of the Great Operations of Surgery* (London: Longman, Hurst, Rees Orme and Brown, 1821)

Bell, J., *The Principles of Surgery* (New York edition: printed by Collins and Perkins, 1810)

Guthrie, G. J., *Commentaries on the Surgery of the War* (London: Henry Renshaw; 1855)

Hennen, J., *Principles of Military Surgery* (Philadelphia edition: Carey & Lea; 1830)

15 G. J. Guthrie, *Commentaries on the Surgery of the War* (London: Henry Renshaw; 1855)

Home, E., *A Treatise on the Blood, Inflammation and Gunshot Wounds*, by the Late John Hunter (London: printed by John Richardson; 1794)

Secondary Sources

Cantlie, N., *A History of the Army Medical Department* (London and Edinburgh: Churchill Livingstone, 1974), Vol. 1
Crumplin, M., *Guthrie's War, a Surgeon of the Peninsula and Waterloo* (Barnsley: Pen & Sword Books Ltd, 2010)
Crumplin, M. K. H. *The Bloody Fields of Waterloo, Medical Support for Wellington's Greatest Battle* (Huntingdon: Ken Trotman Publishing, 2015)
Kaufman, M. H., *The Regius Chair of Military Surgery in the University of Edinburgh 1806–1855* (Amsterdam & New York: Editions Rodopi B.V., 2003)
McGrigor, J., The Tsar's Doctor: The Life and Times of Sir James Wylie (Edinburgh: Birlinn Ltd, 2010)
Moore, Wendy, The *Knife Man* (London: Bantam Press, 2005)

3

Sir James McGrigor

Tom Scotland

Sir James McGrigor (1771–1858) revolutionised medical training in the British Army. In 1971, an editorial in the *Journal of the Royal Army Medical Corps* explained McGrigor`s enduring appeal. He had an intense interest in his profession and took every opportunity to add to his knowledge and skill. He had profound empathy for the common soldier and improved medical care. His integrity, courage and initiative made him well qualified to introduce reforms in the face of opposition. McGrigor led by example, earning the support, loyalty and affection of junior and senior colleagues and practised medicine in a stimulating and congenial environment.[1]

Early Life and Education

James McGrigor was born on 9 April 1771 in the parish of Cromdale, Inverness-shire. His father Colquhoun McGrigor cultivated some land and kept an inn and general merchandise store.[2] Colquhoun McGrigor was ambitious, grew weary scraping a living and moved his family to Aberdeen in 1775, where he set up business as a general merchant.[3]

Scotland at the time was a hub for intellectual and scientific endeavour and achievement in many disciplines and Aberdeen had two universities – King`s College and Marischal College. There were three other Scottish universities at St Andrews, Edinburgh and Glasgow, while England had two, Oxford and Cambridge, which helps explain why so many army medical officers were Scots.

1 Editorial, Sir James McGrigor, 1771–1950, *Journal of the Royal Army Medical Corps,* 117:2 (1971), p.47.

2 Mary McGrigor, *Sir James McGrigor, The Scalpel and the Sword, the Autobiography of the Father of Army Medicine* (Dalkeith: Scottish Cultural Press, 2000), p.13.

3 McGrigor, *Sir James McGrigor, the Scalpel and the Sword,* p.15.

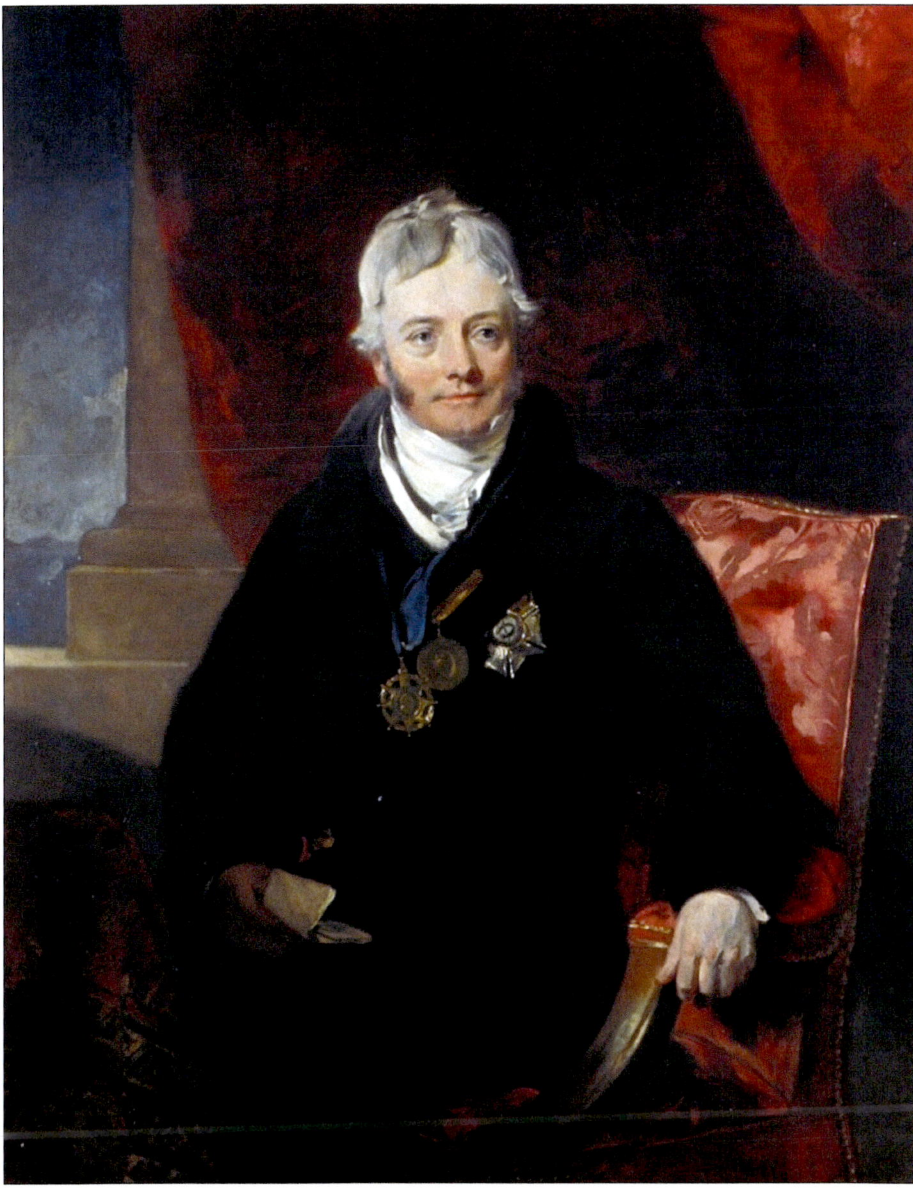

Sir James McGrigor, by Andrew Geddes.
(Collection of the Aberdeen Medico-Chirurgical Society)

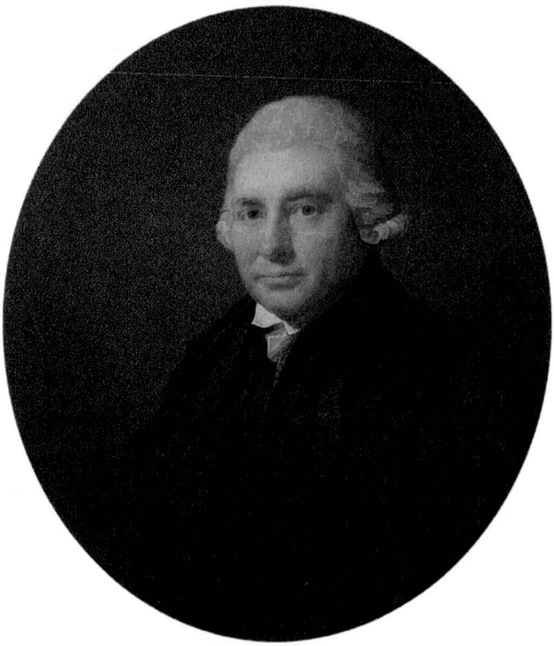

Alexander Monro *secundus* (1733–1817). Stipple engraving by J. Heath, 1880, after Sir Henry Raeburn. (Wellcome Creative Commons Attribution CC BY 4.0 https://creativecommons.org/licences/by/4.0/)

When James was nine, he enrolled at Aberdeen Grammar School and was a very capable and industrious pupil. He learned Latin and Greek for which the school was renowned.[4] He studied classics at Marischal College, graduating *Artium Magister* 'after an examination not the most severe and searching.'[5] Needing more of a challenge, he pursued a career in medicine at Aberdeen Royal Infirmary and was apprenticed to Dr George French (1765–1853), who was also Professor of Chemistry at Marischal College. French was not regarded as a good teacher and was of a decidedly cantankerous nature.[6] McGrigor spent some time in Edinburgh under Alexander Monro *secundus* (1733–1817), anatomist, physician and lecturer in surgery, the second of three generations bearing the name Monro. Like his father before him, Monro *secundus* helped make Edinburgh Medical School a world-famous institute.

In 1789, McGrigor and 11 student colleagues founded the Aberdeen Medical Society as a self-help group because teaching in Aberdeen was poor. They met in homes of parents, where dissertations were delivered. McGrigor was a poor public speaker, being naturally shy. Words sometimes failed him when he made a public address.[7] The society was renamed as the Aberdeen Medico-Chirurgical Society in 1811.

4 J. Gordon, (ed.), *New Statistical Account of Scotland* (Edinburgh: Blackwood, 1845), Vol. XII, pp.43–45.

5 James McGrigor, *Autobiography and Services of Sir James McGrigor, Bart., Late Director General of the Army Medical Department* (London: Longman; 1861), p.3.

6 Alexander Adam, James Hutchison, *The Heritage of the Med-Chi* (Aberdeen: The Medico-Chirurgical Society, 2007), p.22.

7 Adam, Hutchison, *The Heritage of the Med-Chi*, p.4.

Regimental Surgeon

McGrigor left for London in 1793 and after a spell working for an elderly surgeon in Islington, he joined the army. Revolutionary France had declared war on Britain and the Dutch Republic on 1 February 1793. With his father`s help, he purchased a commission as regimental surgeon with the 88th Regiment of Foot, the Connaught Rangers. Not all regimental surgeons were medically qualified and some were barely literate. They were generally despised by serving officers and by army physicians. McGrigor was undeterred. He worked hard and read a great deal, including works by Sir John Pringle,[8] William Cullen,[9] and John Hunter.[10]

In June 1794, the 88th Foot embarked for Jersey where McGrigor contracted typhus fever and was lucky to survive. Regimental surgeons, who were responsible for the care of sick as well as wounded soldiers, often succumbed. Diseases caused four times as many deaths as wounds and were variously attributed to extremes of temperature, soil conditions and miasmata, the foul vapours arising from marshy ground. Epidemic typhus is transmitted by faeces of infected body lice, when scratching allows the infecting organism *Rickettsia Prowazekii* to gain access.

Despite his illness, McGrigor was determined to accompany his regiment when it embarked for Ostend on 28 June to join the Duke of York`s army in the Netherlands. McGrigor recovered and gained valuable experience, treating wounded under heavy enemy fire and on one occasion used a church as a makeshift regimental hospital while a French cannonade pounded the building. 'While engaged in dressing the wounded, I saw several cannon shots go through the walls and some shells burst into the church.'[11]

The expedition ended disastrously in snow and freezing temperatures. Soldiers were inadequately clad and in poor health due to malnutrition and hard drinking. There was an outbreak of typhus and McGrigor was again severely affected. He had to be carried in a cart filled with straw until his ordeal ended when the regiment embarked for England in April 1795.

In November 1795, the regiment joined a force in Portsmouth commanded by Major General Sir Ralph Abercromby (1734–1801) destined for Barbados in the West Indies, where thousands died from mosquito-borne yellow fever and malaria. McGrigor suffered two severe bouts of dysentery and attributed his survival to 'his strong Highland constitution.'[12] In July 1796, orders came for the 88th to return to England and McGrigor occupied his mind by documenting patterns of disease, which he recorded in a subsequent publication.[13]

8 John Pringle, *Observations on the Diseases of the Army* (London: Millar, Wilson & Durham, 1754).
9 William Cullen, *Synopsis Nosologliae Methodicae* (Edinburgh: Murray, 1769).
10 John Hunter, *A Treatise on the Blood, Inflammation and Gun-shot Wounds* (London: Nicol, 1794).
11 McGrigor, *Autobiography*, p.29.
12 McGrigor, *Autobiography*, p.66.
13 James McGrigor, *Medical Sketches of the Expedition to Egypt from India* (London: Murray, 1804).

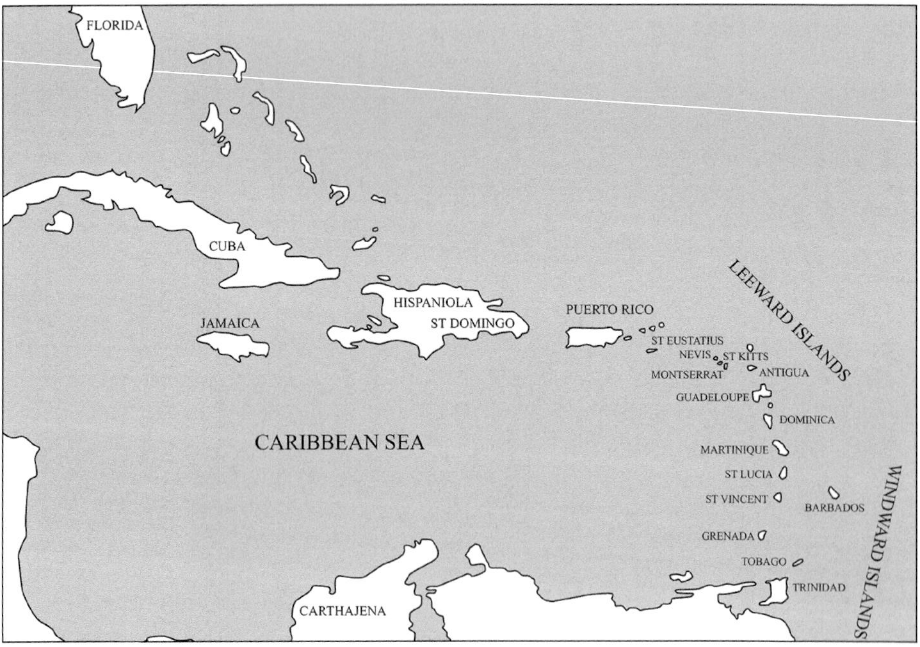

Map of West Indies. (Author`s artwork)

The 88th embarked for India on Christmas Day, 1798 and McGrigor met the then Colonel Arthur Wellesley (1769–1852) for the first time in India. Wellesley was involved in the Siege of Seringapatam, the final act in a war between the East India Company and the Kingdom of Mysore, ruled by Tipu Sultan, the Tiger of Mysore.

McGrigor observed that there had been a great increase in the number of medical officers since the start of the Revolutionary Wars, but not all were well qualified:

> This was occasion of many uneducated and unqualified persons being introduced to the service, not a few of whom, in quarters where the promotion was rapid, found means to pass through different grades to the rank of regimental and staff surgeon.[14]

Determined to maintain his own high standards, McGrigor submitted a summary of his detailed records made between 1 June 1800 and 31 May 1801 to the *Edinburgh Medical and Surgical Journal.* His findings were published in 1805.[15]

14 McGrigor, *Autobiography*, pp.93–94.

15 James McGrigor, *A Memoir on the State of Health of the 88th Regiment, and of the Corps attached to it, from 1st June 1800 to 31st May 1801, as originally presented to the Medical Board of Bombay, in The Edinburgh Medical and Surgical Journal, exhibiting a concise view of the latest and most important developments in medicine, surgery and pharmacy, Vol. I* (Edinburgh: Archibald Constable and Company, 1805).

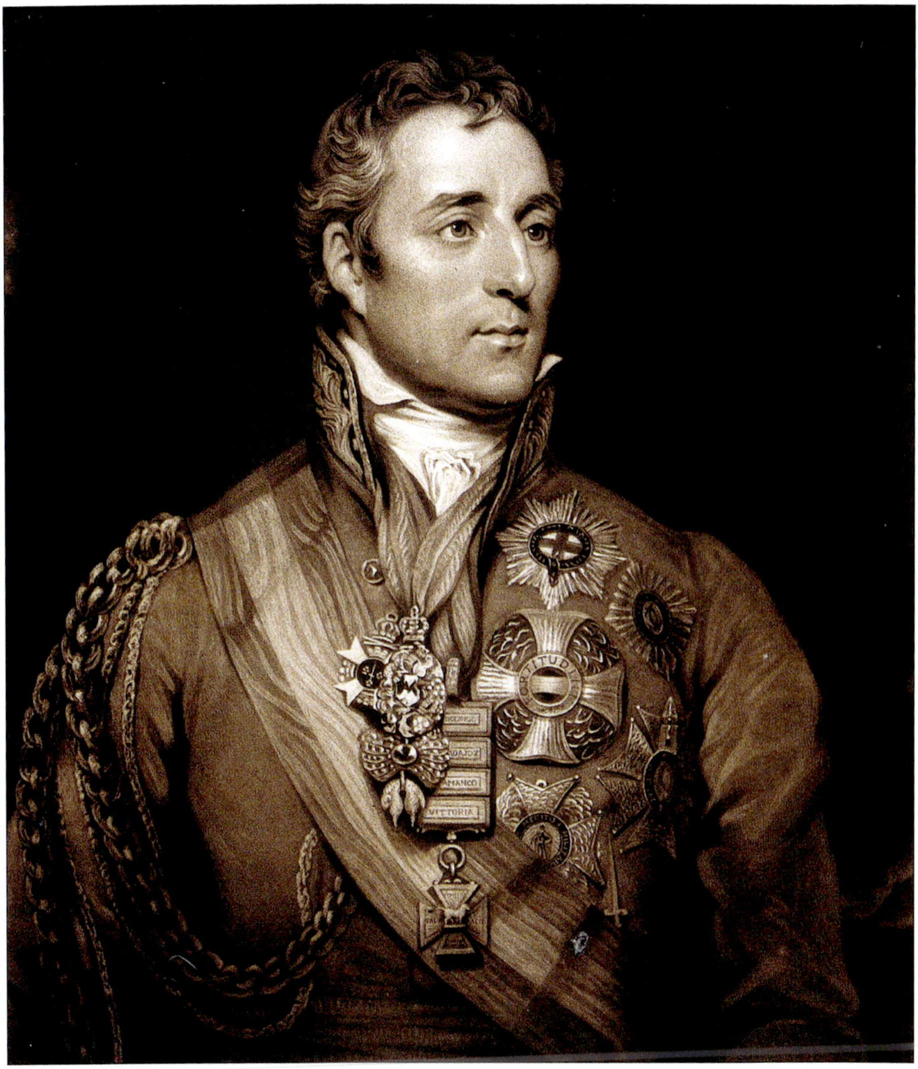

Arthur Wellesley, 1st Duke of Wellington, mezzotint by W. Say 1814, after T. Phillips. (Wellcome Collection; Public Domain https://wellcomecollection.org/works/wkavzcwe)

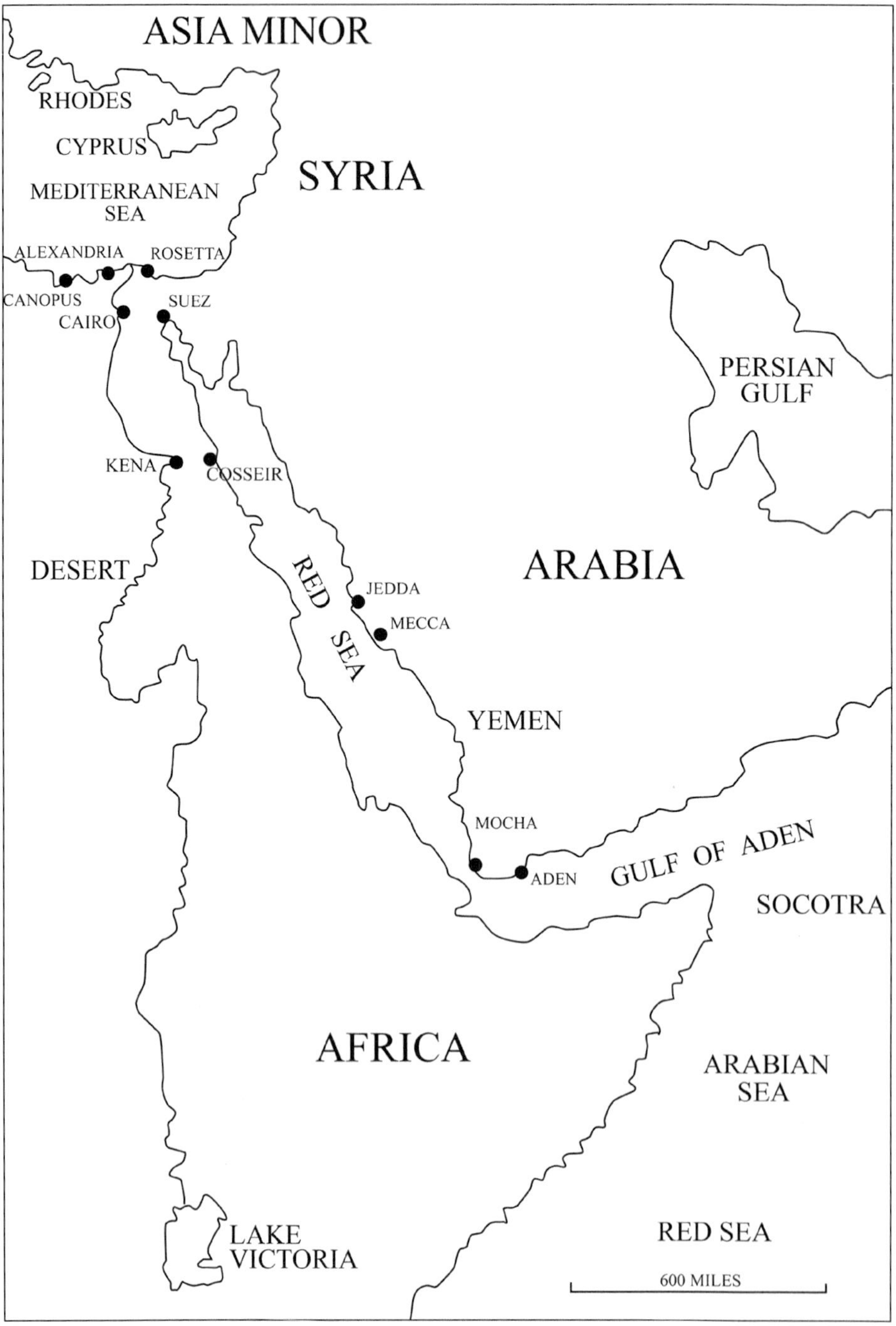

Map of Egypt and Arabia. (Author`s artwork)

Egypt, and in Charge of Medical Services

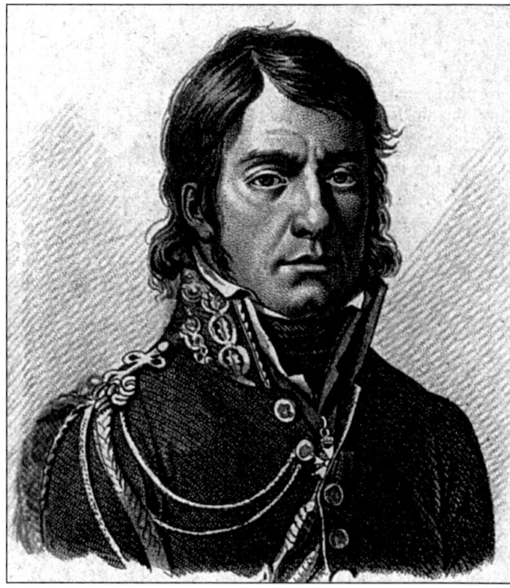

Dominique Jean, Baron Larrey, stipple engraving by A. Tardieu after himself. (Wellcome Collection, Licence: Creative Commons Attribution CC BY 4.0) https://creativecommons.org/licenses/by/4.0/)

On 3 April 1801, the 88th joined a combined force of British and East India Company regiments under the command of General Sir David Baird (1757–1829) to assist the army of Sir Ralph Abercromby in expelling the French forces from Egypt. The French, under Bonaparte had invaded in 1798, but Nelson's victory at the Battle of the Nile (1/2 August 1798) had stranded the French. Bonaparte soon returned to France, leaving his army behind. McGrigor was in charge of medical services, 'the first King's medical officer who was ever so employed in a joint venture.'[16] He formed a good rapport with Baird and considered prevention of disease of the utmost importance. 'A good commanding officer has, in general, a healthy regiment. Everything can be done in the prevention of disease, but unfortunately, very little in the treatment when it supervenes.'[17] McGrigor cultivated symbiotic relationships with commanding officers, making it easier to introduce preventive measures.[18] He dealt with an outbreak of bubonic plague in Egypt which had first affected French soldiers. He also encountered a condition called Egyptian Ophthalmia, which could cause blindness, and was probably caused by a variety of organisms including Koch-Week's bacillus (otherwise known as *Haemophylis aegyptius*), *Gonococcus* and *Chlamydia trachoma*.[19] Some cases were probably self-inflicted.[20]

16 McGrigor. *Autobiography*, pp.106–107.
17 James McGrigor, *Medical Sketches of the Expedition to Egypt from India.* (London: Murray, 1804), p.95.
18 C. Kelly, Medicine and the Egyptian Campaign: The Development of the Military Medical Officer during the Napoleonic Wars, *Canadian Bulletin of Medical History*, 27: 2 (2010), pp.321–342.
19 M. Meyerhof, 'A Short History of Ophthalmia during the Egyptian Campaign of 1798–1807' in *British Journal of Ophthalmology*, 16 (March 1932), pp.129–152.
20 William Fergusson, *Notes and Recollections of a Professional Life* (London: Longman, Brown, Green and Longmans, 1846), pp.110–112.

In September 1801, French forces surrendered Alexandria and McGrigor met Baron Dominique Larrey (1766–1842), Bonaparte's Chief Medical Officer. They formed a lasting friendship and in 1817, Larrey became an Honorary Member of the Aberdeen Medico-Chirurgical Society.[21]

Deputy Inspector of Hospitals

In February 1804, McGrigor transferred briefly to the Royal Regiment of Horse Guards (Blue) and was awarded the degree of MD by Marischal College for his thesis *The Merits of Regimental Hospitals.* His organisational skills soon led to his appointment as Deputy Inspector of Hospitals for the Northern District in June 1805. Based in Beverley, he was in his element:

> My appointment was one which was particularly congenial to my mind and habits. From my first entrance into the service I had some turn for statistical statements, for collecting medical facts and generalising upon them, and I made, for my own satisfaction monthly, quarterly and annual statements of the diseases which had come under my notice.[22]

In 1838, data collected by McGrigor would be used by Scottish military statistician Henry Marshall (1775–1851) to dismiss many of the misperceptions regarding the aetiology of diseases.[23]

In June 1806, McGrigor was promoted to Deputy Inspector of Hospitals for the South-West District. Based at Winchester, it was the busiest such post in the country:

> My charge was now the greatest in the country, for besides the great number of troops, I had the harassing duties of embarkations and disembarkations at Portsmouth; and furthermore the large general hospital at the Isle of Wight; with the great depot for Ophthalmia and other ocular diseases, often containing 1,000 cases of diseases of the eye.[24]

In January 1809, McGrigor dealt with sick and wounded soldiers of the late Sir John Moore`s army, evacuated from Corunna in Spain. Moore himself had been killed at the Battle of Corunna on 16 January. McGrigor described conditions when troop ships arrived in Portsmouth:

21 J. S. Riddel, *The Records of the Aberdeen Medico-Chirurgical Society from 1789 to 1922* (Aberdeen: W&W Lindsay, 1922), p.78.
22 McGrigor, *Autobiography*, pp.177–178.
23 Henry Marshall, *Statistical report on the sickness, mortality, and invaliding among the troops in the West Indies* (London: Clowes and Sons for Her Majesty`s Stationery Office, 1838).
24 McGrigor, *Autobiography*, p.211.

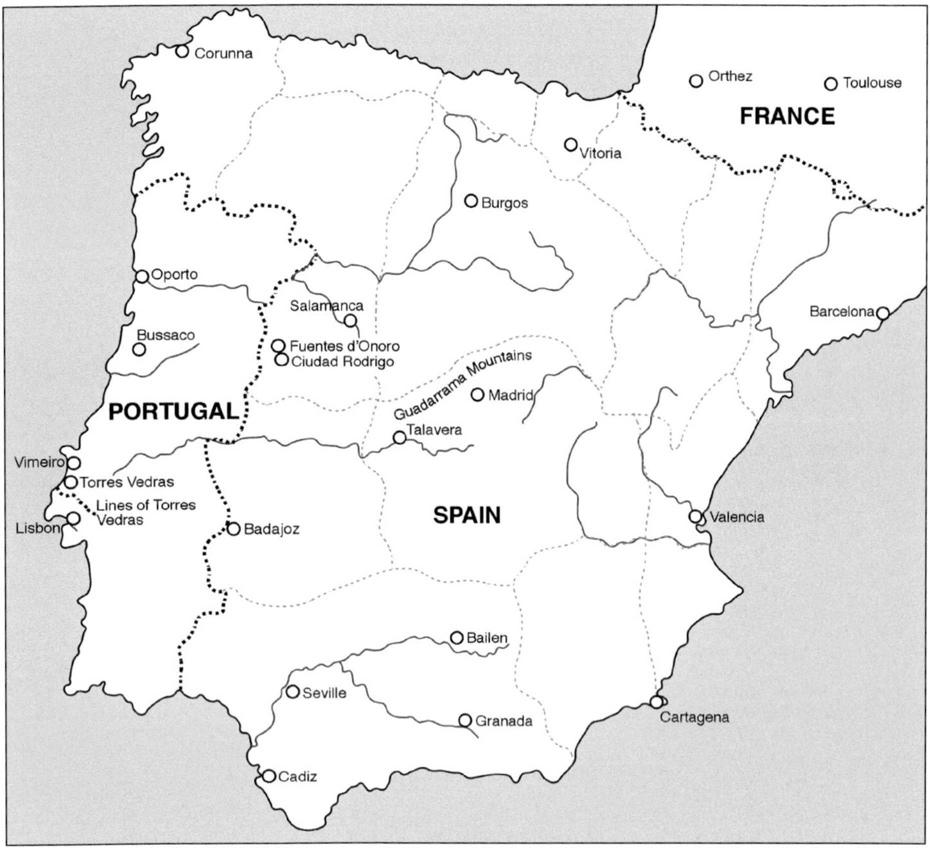

Map of Spain and Portugal. (Gordon Sables, Department of Medical Illustration, University of Aberdeen)

> By the time they disembarked, typhus fever had spread widely among them. Never was situation more favourable for the propagation of contagion than the mode of return of the British from Corunna.[25]

On 9 April 1809, Sir Arthur Wellesley landed in Lisbon to command an Anglo-Portuguese army. He became Viscount Wellington after the Battle of Talavera on 27 July 1809. Despite this and other subsequent successes, Wellington became concerned by the large numbers of sick in his army. Many were veterans of a campaign on 30 July 1809 to the island of Walcheren, now part of the reclaimed land mass of The Netherlands. The aim had been to capture Antwerp and relieve

25 McGrigor, *Autobiography*, pp.215–216.

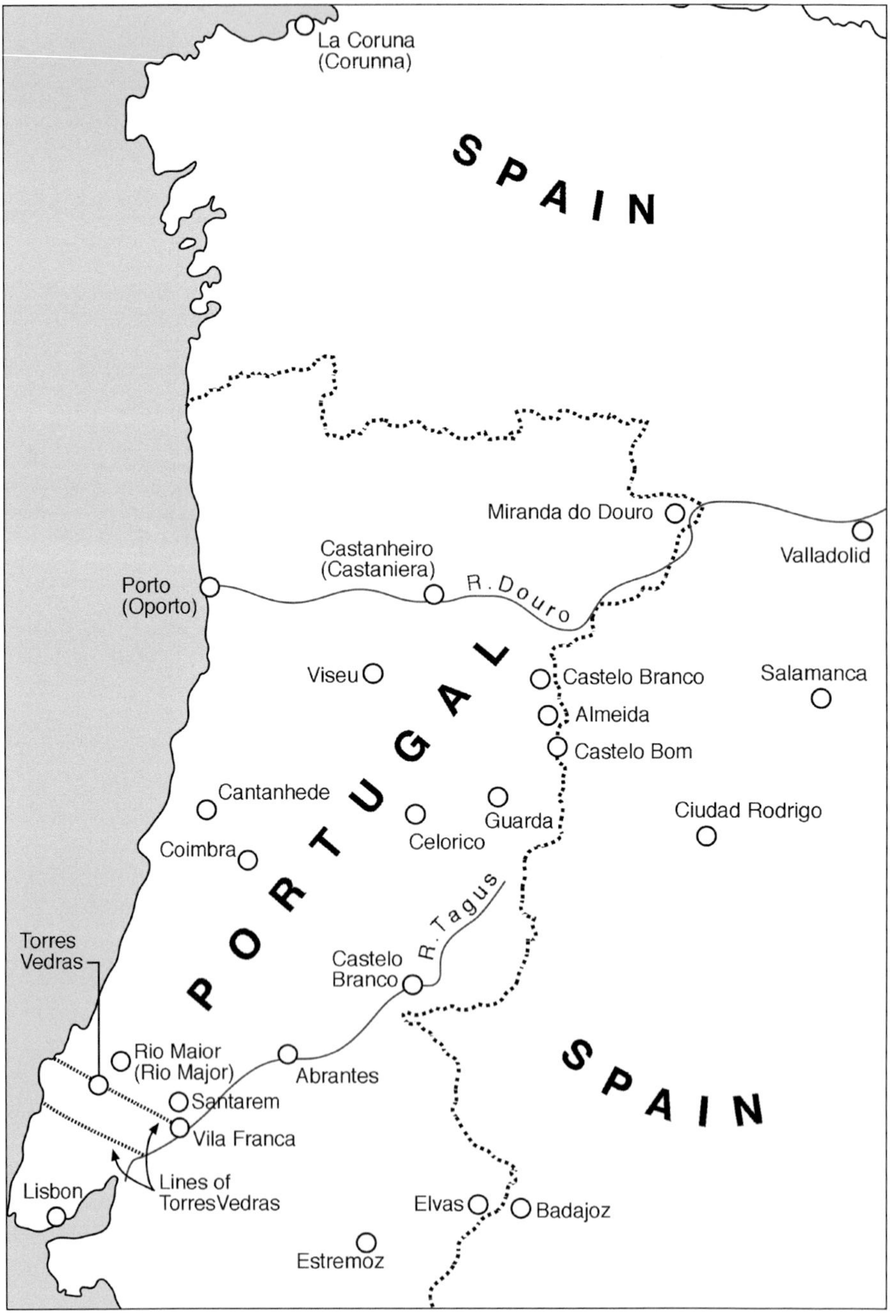

Detailed Map of Portugal. (Gordon Stables; Department of Medical Illustration, University of Aberdeen)

pressure on the Austrian allies in the Fifth Coalition, but Austria had already been defeated by Napoleon at Wagram on 5/6 July 1809. By December 1809, no fewer than 4,000 soldiers from a force of 40,000 had died of 'Walcheren Fever', probably a lethal cocktail of typhus, typhoid, malaria and dysentery.[26] 11,000 survived, chronically sick, many of whom went to the Peninsula. Others in the Peninsular army were raw recruits in poor health from the outset and not acclimatised. In a dispatch to Horse Guards dated 3 October 1811 Wellington requested that, 'to replace Dr Franck, who was ill, he should have the most active and intelligent person that can be found to fill his place.'[27]

Inspector General of Hospitals

McGrigor reached Lisbon in January 1812 as Inspector General of Hospitals. He immediately made improvements in the apothecary and purveyor departments. There were many apparently sick officers at Belem and other convalescent depots being cared for by a disproportionately large number of medical officers.[28] McGrigor sent many to join Wellington, who would soon besiege the border fortress of Badajoz. McGrigor himself set off to join his Commander in Chief via general hospitals in Portugal, making improvements as he went. At Coimbra he segregated sick from wounded and established convalescent hospitals. Too many sick were dying from relapses of disease after being discharged directly to cold barracks. At Celorico, he improved cleanliness and ventilation of hospitals.[29] He was convinced it would be better to expand regimental hospitals close to the fighting and send as few as possible to distant general hospitals. Those with minor conditions would return to duty more quickly, while seriously sick and wounded would be spared potentially life-threatening journeys in unsprung bullock carts to general hospitals in Portugal. The French had a much better evacuation system. Larrey`s *'ambulance volante'*, comprising three divisions, each with 113 men and each equipped with eight light and four heavy sprung wagons, removed wounded soldiers directly from the battlefield.[30] Wellington refused to sanction the use of good transport to evacuate sick and wounded and was reluctant to develop regimental hospitals.

After the Battle of Salamanca on 22 July 1812, McGrigor announced he had used good transport to evacuate the wounded. Wellington flew into a fit of rage and roared:

26 M. R. Howard, 'Walcheren 1809: A Medical Catastrophe' in *British Medical Journal*, 319:7225 (London: 1999), pp.1642–1645.
27 D. G. McGrigor, 'Sir James McGrigor; some notes and correspondence' in *Journal of the Royal Army Medical Corps*, 96:1 (London: 1951), pp.56–63.
28 McGrigor, *Autobiography*, p.256.
29 McGrigor, *Sir James McGrigor*, *The Scalpel and the Sword*, pp.169–170.
30 Robert Richardson, *Larrey: Surgeon to Napoleon`s Imperial Guard* (London: John Murray Ltd., 1974), pp.34–37.

> I shall be glad to know who is to command this army, I or you. I establish one route, one line of communication for the army; you establish another, and order the commissariat by that line. As long as you live, sir, never do that again; never do anything without my orders.[31]

Wellington`s anger soon subsided and he invited McGrigor to dinner.

In October 1812, Wellington was besieging Burgos near Madrid where the campaign was going badly. He summoned McGrigor and said: 'I must leave this place this very night. But what is to become of our sick and wounded?' [32] McGrigor replied that he had used the carts and mules that came up with provisions for the army to send back every one that could be moved to the hospitals which he had established.[33] So began the retreat into Portugal of an army which had become a hungry, cold, demoralised and drunken rabble, and there were outbreaks of typhus and dysentery.

McGrigor successfully transformed the army`s health over the winter of 1812/1813. He persuaded Wellington to make full use of regimental hospitals, increasing their total capacity from 2,000 to 5,000. Fewer seriously sick were evacuated in unsprung bullock carts. 'In a short time the march of sick to the established hospitals in the rear was stopped; and it was high time, for the number that died on the way, of those sent to the rear was great.'[34] Early supportive measures in regimental hospitals probably improved prognosis of those who were seriously sick and less severely affected individuals quickly returned to duty. McGrigor arranged for prefabricated hospital and barrack accommodation to be brought from Britain. He ensured that soldiers received fresh clothing and blankets and were provided with a bedstead to lie on rather than straw. Good provisions improved nutritional status. Thanks partly to McGrigor, the Battle of Vitoria on 21 June 1813 was an overwhelming victory for Wellington:

> It was said with much truth by an eminent individual, that he thought the extraordinary exertions of the medical officers of the army might be said to have decided the day at Vitoria, for their exertions had undoubtedly added a full division in strength to Lord Wellington`s army, and without these 4,000 or 5,000 men, it is more than doubtful if his lordship, with all his unrivalled talents, could have carried the day.[35]

Arthur Butler, author of the *Official History of Australian Medical Services during the Great War* wrote: 'Sir James McGrigor was master of the technique "return to duty", with whose help in the Peninsular War Wellington brought the organisation and working of the medical services to a pitch of perfection till then unapproached in any

31 McGrigor, *Autobiography*, p.202.
32 McGrigor, *Autobiography*, p.306.
33 McGrigor, *Autobiography*, p.307.
34 McGrigor, *Autobiography*, p.324.
35 McGrigor, *Autobiography*, p.331.

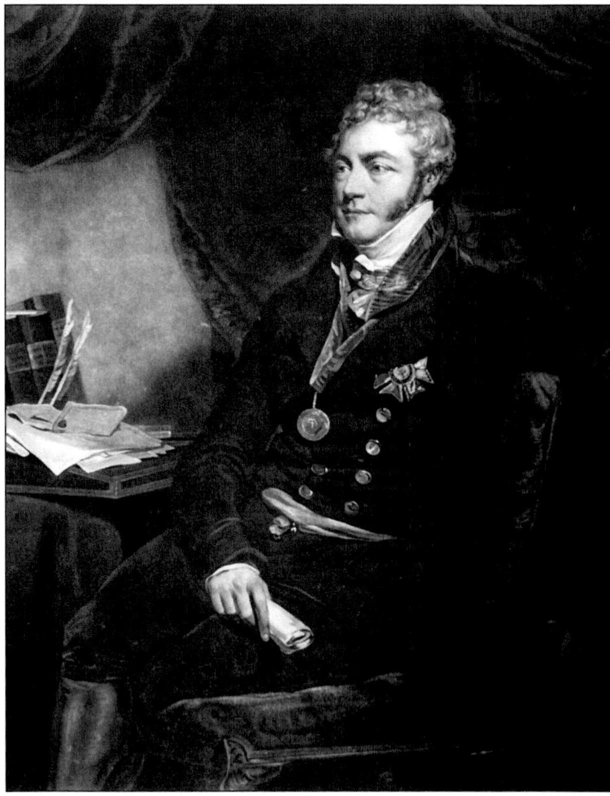

Sir James McGrigor, mezzotint by W. Ward after Jackson. Portrait painted late 1810s to early 1820s. (Wellcome Collection Creative Commons Attribution CC BY 4.0https://creativecommons.org/licenses/by/4.0/>)

European army.'[36] British casualties at Vitoria were 501 killed and 2,807 wounded.[37] Surgeons dealt with Spanish, Portuguese and captured French wounded. McGrigor was responsible for ensuring surgeons were well trained. He instructed senior medical officers to submit confidential reports on ability and application of medical officers under their supervision. Diaries and casebooks were submitted as evidence. McGrigor was a fierce critic of any who did not pull his weight. George James Guthrie (1785–1856) was Wellington`s most famous surgeon and McGrigor quickly realised how good Guthrie was, declaring, 'He and I must be friends.'[38] McGrigor wrote, 'Great experience had at this time created among us a body of operators such as never were excelled, if ever before equalled in the British Army.'[39]

36 A. G. Butler, *Official History of the Australian Army Medical Services 1914–1918, Volume II – The Western Front* (Canberra: Australian War Memorial, 1940), p.483.
37 D. Smith, *The Greenhill Napoleonic Wars Data Book* (London: Lionel Leventhal Limited, 1998), p.426.
38 Michael Crumplin, *Guthrie`s War* (Barnsley: Pen and Sword Books Ltd., 2010), p.78.
39 McGrigor, *Autobiography*, p.340.

Director General of Army Medical Services

James McGrigor became Director General of Army Medical Services on 13 June 1815 and remained in post until 1850. His aim was to provide the best possible medical care for the common soldier. He wrote:

> Whatever may formerly have been the condition of those who entered the medical department of the army, it is now, and has been, far otherwise, for the last 30 or 40 years at least. Moral character is investigated in every candidate, and the qualifications required of each are of a very high order; indeed more is now required of each candidate for the army than is required for civil life by either of the colleges of physicians or surgeons of London, Edinburgh and Dublin[40]

James McGrigor died in London on 2 April 1858 and was buried in Kensal Green Cemetery, London.

Bibliography

Books

Adam, A., Hutchison, J., *The Heritage of the Med-Chi* (Aberdeen: The Medico-Chirurgical Society, 2007)

Butler, A.G., *Official History of the Australian Army Medical Services 1914–1918, Volume II – The Western Front* (Canberra: Australian War Memorial, 1940)

Crumplin, M., *Guthrie's War* (Barnsley: Pen and Sword Books Ltd., 2010)

Cullen, W., *Synopsis Nosologliae Methodicae* (Edinburgh: Murray, 1769)

Fergusson, W., *Notes and Recollections of a Professional Life* (London: Longman, Brown, Green and Longmans, 1846).

Gordon, J. (ed.), *New Statistical Account of Scotland, Vol. XII* (Edinburgh: Blackwood, 1845)

Hunter, J., *A Treatise on the Blood, Inflammation and Gun-shot Wounds* (London: Nicol, 1794)

Marshall, Henry, Statistical *Report on the Sickness, Mortality, and Invaliding Among the Troops in the West Indies* (London: Clowes and Sons for Her Majesty's Stationery Office, 1838)

McGrigor, J., *A Memoir on the State of Health of the 88th Regiment, and of the Corps attached to it, from 1st June 1800 to 31st May 1801, as originally presented to the Medical Board of Bombay, in The Edinburgh Medical and Surgical Journal, exhibiting a concise view of the latest and most important developments in medicine, surgery and pharmacy, Vol. I* (Edinburgh: Archibald Constable and Company, 1805)

40 McGrigor, *Autobiography*, p.197

McGrigor, J., *Autobiography and Services of Sir James McGrigor, Bart., Late Director General of the Army Medical Department* (London: Longman, 1861)
McGrigor, J., *Medical Sketches of the Expedition to Egypt from India* (London: Murray, 1804)
McGrigor, M., *Sir James McGrigor, The Scalpel and the Sword, the Autobiography of the Father of Army Medicine* (Dalkeith: Scottish Cultural Press; 2000)
Pringle, J., *Observations on the Diseases of the Army* (London: Millar, Wilson & Durham, 1754)
Richardson, R., *Larrey: Surgeon to Napoleon's Imperial Guard* (London: John Murray Ltd., 1974)
Riddel, J.S., *The Records of the Aberdeen Medico-Chirurgical Society from 1789 to 1922* (Aberdeen: W&W Lindsay, 1922)
Smith, Digby, *The Greenhill Napoleonic Wars Data Book* (London: Lionel Leventhal Limited, 1998)

Journals

Editorial, Sir James McGrigor, 1771–1950, *Journal of the Royal Army Medical Corps,* 117:2 (London: 1971), p.47
Howard, M. R., 'Walcheren 1809: A Medical Catastrophe' in *British Medical Journal*, 319:7225 (London: 1999), pp.1642–1645
Kelly, C., 'Medicine and the Egyptian Campaign: The Development of the Military Medical Officer during the Napoleonic Wars' in *Canadian Bulletin of Medical History*, 27: 2 (Toronto: 2010), pp.321–342
McGrigor, D. G., 'Sir James McGrigor; some notes and correspondence' in *Journal Royal Army Medical Corps*, 96:1 (London: 1951), pp.56–63.
Meyerhof, M., 'A Short History of Ophthalmia during the Egyptian Campaign of 1798–1807' in *British Journal of Ophthalmology*, 16, March 1932 (London:1932), pp.129–152

4

Scottish Physicians and Surgeons of Nelson's Navy

Peter Brinsden

Introduction

Few living today can imagine the carnage that existed during sea battles in the ships of the Royal Navy in the time of Nelson. Sailors were raked by cannon, grapeshot, musket balls and lethal flying wood splinters – all amongst the din and clamour, dense gunpowder smoke, screaming of the wounded and blood-soaked decks. There can have been no greater hell than that experienced by the officers and men manning the great wooden battleships of Nelson's navy.

The ship's surgeon would have been in his own little hell; stationed on the orlop deck – below the main deck and below the waterline – in a dark, fetid sickbay, with the thunderous rumble and roar of cannon firing on the deck above him. He would push his hard-honed surgical skills, deep knowledge of anatomy and trauma care to their extremes. His patients would have been sitting and lying around on the deck close by moaning, screaming, bleeding and dying. They were taken to the surgeon in strict order from the time they were brought down to the sickbay – officers and seamen together.

Having painted this gruesome picture, it should be appreciated that surgery in action situations in fact played a very small part in the life of a ship's surgeon. It has been estimated that only about five percent of a surgeon's time was spent in action, with only 1.5 percent of all seamen who died during the Napoleonic Wars dying in battle. Twelve percent of his work resulted from wreck, fire and explosions. The vast majority – 85 percent of deaths in the Royal Navy during the Revolutionary and Napoleonic Wars with France (1792–1815) were due to disease and accidents.[1] The surgeon was, therefore, a surgeon, a physician and an apothecary. During this period the Royal Navy suffered almost continuous lethal epidemics of dysentery, typhus,

1 David McLean, *Surgeons of the Fleet* (London: Tauris, 2010), p.1.

scurvy, malaria and yellow fever. The annual death rate in the Navy was about 1 in 42 in 1779, but this reduced quite dramatically to 1 in 143 by 1813, largely due to improvements in medical care.

Despite frequent and not very flattering tales of drunkenness and bad behaviour, the ship's surgeon was respected and usually skilled as a surgical technician, with a deep knowledge of human anatomy and, importantly, an appreciation of the need for speed in operating. This was critical to the chance of a patient surviving from the shock of amputation and other major trauma surgery. Post-operative infection was expected, from inflammation leading to 'laudable pus' and potentially, and often ultimately, to gangrene and finally to death.

Most medical care in Britain's Royal Navy was provided by ships' surgeons. There were a few naval physicians who were qualified medical practitioners. These were generally better educated and of a higher social class than surgeons – and were more honoured and therefore better paid. In 1775, for example, there were only three qualified physicians in the Navy. Although better qualified, the treatments often provided by physicians included brandy enemas, strychnine injections, sulphuric acid gargles, ammonia applied to the lips, and bleeding to treat pneumonia. We now know that none of these treatments actually worked, unlike the efforts of the naval surgeon generally. Interestingly, pay scales, for example in the year of 1805, gave a surgeon's daily rate of pay after 10 years of active service at just 14 shillings a day, or £255/10 per annum, which equates today to about £18,500. Physicians, on the other hand, received 29 shillings per day, equivalent to £529 per annum, the equivalent of which today is £38,500. Nevertheless, the usefulness of a ship's surgeon on a day-to-day basis was much greater than that of a physician at that time. Some physicians, however, were often able to see the 'bigger picture' when it came to the discovery of the causes and potential remedies for the biggest killers of seamen like scurvy, malaria, typhus et cetera, as discussed elsewhere in this book.

Scottish Surgeons and Physicians

As background, it is interesting to note the relative populations of the United Kingdom in the early nineteenth century: 57 percent of the total UK population was from England and Wales, 33 percent from Ireland and just 10 percent from Scotland. What is striking is the disproportionate number of Scottish surgeons and physicians in the Royal Navy during the period of the Revolutionary and Napoleonic Wars, in comparison with the proportion of Scots in the total population of the United Kingdom. That 10 percent of the population should produce between 45 and 60 percent of Royal Naval surgeons and physicians at that time is remarkable.

Looking in more detail at where Scottish naval surgeons originated from – some 50 percent were from 12 different Scottish counties and the remaining 50 percent were from Perth and Aberdeen; only two of 29 were from Edinburgh. Data from the National Archives (ADM 48), show the family backgrounds of Scottish naval surgeons at the time. 15 of 40 were from the professions, including half from families in the medical profession; 5 of 40 were from agricultural backgrounds while others included 8 from merchant families, labourers, builders and tradesmen.[2]

Most surgical apprentices in the late eighteenth and early nineteenth century would have started their apprenticeships between the age of 14 and 16 years, but some are known to have started as early as 13. They would have worked with general practitioners and local surgeons in Scotland and later applied for positions with the Royal Navy, then passing through an interview and examination process.

Physicians from Scotland who trained at the University of Edinburgh were required to pass written and oral examinations in Latin and they had to defend their theses in Latin as well; at the time Latin was the language of international scientific discourse.

The competition for positions in civilian practice for both surgeons and physicians in Scotland was fierce, as it also was in London and Dublin. Without connections and patronage, the chances of a good job were close to nil. The Navy and the Army therefore offered newly trained physicians and surgeons opportunities, saving them from probable unemployment.

Some of the best available data on the demography of Royal Naval surgeons are to be found in an article in the *Journal of World-Historical Information* by Christopher Myers. Myers shows the country of origin of naval surgeons and the universities where they had trained between the years 1795 and 1829, which covers the period of the Revolutionary and Napoleonic Wars. His data show that some 45 percent of all ranks of physicians or surgeons came from the University of Edinburgh, compared to only 25 percent from English medical schools.[3] It bears being reminded that Scotland only accounted for 10 percent of the population of the United Kingdom at the time.

In an excellent review entitled 'Scotland, Scottishness, British Integration and the Royal Navy, 1793 to 1815', Dr Sarah Caputo states that 'the "Scottish connection" with the Royal Navy was prominent'. In addition to surgeons and physicians, Scotland also produced some of the best-known naval officers, including Adam Duncan, the victor of Camperdown (1797), George Keith Elphinstone, who conquered the Cape of Good Hope in 1795, and Thomas Cochran, 10th Earl of Dundonald, a renowned frigate captain.[4]

The quality of medical care in His Majesty's Royal Navy ships improved greatly during the time of the Wars, thanks largely to the efforts of a number of prominent Scottish naval surgeons and physicians, including Dr James Lind, who is often regarded as the father of modern naval medicine.

2 David B Haycock and Sally Archer, *Health & Medicine at Sea 1700–1900* (Woodbridge: Boydell Press, 2009), p.42.

3 Christopher H. Myers, 'The Demography of Royal Naval Surgeons: Some views on the Process of Prosopography' in *Journal of World-Historical Information*, 2–3 (Pittsburgh: 2014–2015), pp.43–53.

4 Sarah Caputo, 'Scotland, Scottishness, British Integration and the Royal Navy, 1793 to 1815' in *The Scottish Historical Review*, 97.1 (Edinburgh: 2018), pp.85–118.

Celebrated Scottish Surgeons and Physicians who served in the Era of Nelson's Navy

Dr James Lind (1716–1794)

James Lind was educated at Edinburgh University, where he is celebrated with a plaque extolling him as "the Hippocrates of naval medicine". He served as a ship's surgeon between 1739 and 1748 and published extensively on medical conditions at sea. In 1761, he even devised a system for distilling drinkable water on board ships. In 1763 he published a paper on fevers and infections on board ship. However, he is most famous for having conducted the world's first ever clinical trial while he was on board HMS *Salisbury*. He proved that oranges and lemons can cure, and also prevent, the dreaded (at the time mainly maritime) disease of scurvy. He published his famous *Treatise on Scurvy* in 1753. This discovery, sadly, upset many of his jealous and sceptical more senior colleagues, and delayed the routine issue of lemon juice for another 42 years. He was promoted to the role of senior physician at RNH (Royal Naval Hospital) *Haslar* shortly after publication, serving there for the next 25 years.

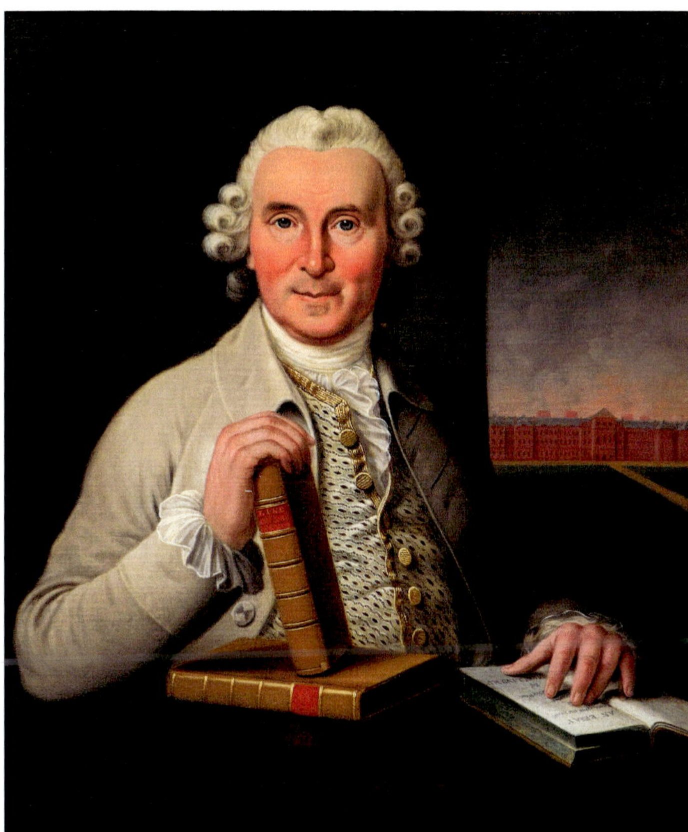

James Lind, by George Chalmers. (Copyright John Hepner, reproduced with permission)

It bears remembering that scurvy was one of the greatest causes of sickness and death among officers and men of the eighteenth and early nineteenth century navies. It invariably followed long sea voyages, during which there would be a complete lack of fresh meat, vegetables, and fruit. It is, of course, now well known that scurvy is caused by a deficiency in the diet of vitamin C, the identity of which was not discovered until long after Lind's treatise was published. The symptoms and signs of scurvy are multiple and include: malaise and lethargy; dyspnoea (shortness of breath); muscle and bone pain; gum disease and loosening of the teeth; a tendency to bruising and skin rashes; the failure of wounds to heal; and sometimes severe emotional changes. Late changes include severe oedema (swelling), oliguria (poor urine output), neuropathy (nerve damage), fever, convulsions and, finally, death. Ultimately Lind may have been responsible for preserving the health and saving the lives of more men in the Royal Navy than the instigator of any other medical intervention or treatment in its history, thus helping to preserve Britain's world supremacy at sea until the early twentieth century.

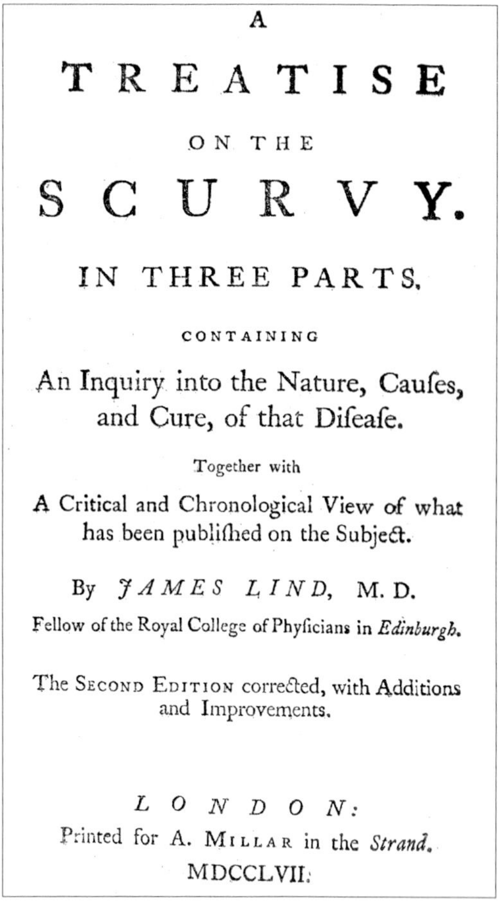

A

TREATISE

ON THE

SCURVY.

IN THREE PARTS.

CONTAINING

An Inquiry into the Nature, Cauſes, and Cure, of that Diſeaſe.

Together with

A Critical and Chronological View of what has been publiſhed on the Subject.

By *JAMES LIND*, M. D.

Fellow of the Royal College of Phyſicians in *Edinburgh*.

The SECOND EDITION corrected, with Additions and Improvements.

LONDON:

Printed for A. MILLAR in the *Strand*.

MDCCLVII.

Frontispiece to Lind's Treatise on the Scurvy. (Wellcome collection. CC BY 4.0 Attribution 4.0)

Surgeon Vice Admiral Sir James Watt, Medical Director General, Royal Navy (1972–1977), in an article in the *Journal of the Royal Society of Medicine* stated:

> James Lind was perhaps the greatest of all naval surgeons, and his death in comparative obscurity illustrates the fate of highly original thinkers dependent upon powerful and unperceptive patrons. It was 48 years after he had conclusively demonstrated that lemon and orange juice would cure and prevent scurvy before a reluctant Admiralty could be persuaded to make a general issue to the Fleet. That was only because the more socially acceptable Sir Gilbert Blane endorsed Lind's work. Within two years, scurvy had virtually disappeared, and Carré (1976), the French medical historian, believes that Lind, by providing British

admirals with fit men, contributed decisively to Napoleon's defeat. Typhus was similarly eliminated by Lind's measures, and the incidence of malaria and yellow fever drastically reduced by his preventive proposals.[5]

While this presents an over-optimistic view of the elimination of typhus, Lind made important contributions to the prevention of disease in the Royal Navy as did two other later Scots, the army physician Robert Jackson (1750–1827) and the naval surgeon Archibald Menzies (1754–1842).[6]

Dr Gilbert Blane (1749–1834)

Gilbert Blane – later to become Sir Gilbert Blane of Blanefield, 1st Baronet, MD FRCSEd MRCP FRS – studied medicine at Edinburgh and graduated MD from Glasgow University in 1778. He was a Scottish physician who instituted many health reforms in the Royal Navy and achieved the position of Physician to the Fleet from 1779 to 1883. He published several medical papers, one of the most important of which was titled, *On the most effective means for preserving the health of seamen, particularly in the Royal Navy*. He finally introduced lemon juice (later replaced by limes), as a daily addition to the naval diet in 1795 – 42 years after Lind had advocated it! In 1795 Blane was appointed Commissioner of the Sick and Hurt Board of the Admiralty, during which time he went to great lengths to ensure the provision to all sailors of soap, lemons, proper victualling and proper ventilation of living spaces on board HM ships. He also advocated the issue to each Royal Navy sailor of a tourniquet to stem catastrophic bleeding in battle.

In his role as the Commissioner of the Sick and Hurt Board, he introduced mandatory seven years of training for all naval surgeons, followed by an examination to prove their competence prior to being appointed. On his return to Britain following his time with the Mediterranean Fleet, he became a physician to Saint Thomas's Hospital from 1783 to 1795, Physician Extraordinary to the Prince of Wales in 1786 and Physician in Ordinary to King George IV, and later to King William IV. He was made Baronet Blanefield in 1812.

Blane is still well remembered within the Royal Naval Medical Service as having established a fund for the encouragement of naval medical science. The fund of £300 was to be used to confirm gold medals to the medical officer of the Royal Navy who was judged to have demonstrated, 'the most distinguished proofs of skill, diligence, humanity and learning in the exercise of their professional duties.'[7] The Gilbert

5 James Watt, 'Some Forgotten Contributions of Naval Surgeons' in *Journal of the Royal Society of Medicine*. 78:9 (London: 1985), pp.753–762.

6 Chelsea Chan and Andreas Demetriades, 'The Contributions of James Carmichael Smyth, Archibald Menzies and Robert Jackson to the Treatment of Typhus in Royal Naval Vessels in the Late 18th Century' in *Journal of Medical Biography*. 31;1 (London: 2023) pp.4–9.

7 J. G. Penn-Barwell, 'Sir Gilbert Blane FRS: The Man and his Legacy' in *Journal of the Royal Naval Medical Service* 102 (London: 2016) pp.61–66.

Blane Medal is still awarded annually, alternately by the Royal College of Surgeons of England and the Royal College of Physicians, upon the recommendation of the Medical Director General (Navy).

Dr John Snipe (? –1805)

John Snipe, a Scottish physician, was the first physician to be appointed to Admiral Lord Nelson's Mediterranean Fleet in 1804. There, like Gilbert Blane, he emphasised that strict attention to hygiene of sailors was mandatory, that clothing for all seasons should be issued to the sailors, that their accommodation should be clean and dry and that there should be suitable accommodation for the sick; also, that they should have a nourishing diet. He argued that the health of the Fleet hinged on close cooperation between a ship's senior officers and the medical establishment. Admiral Nelson is quoted at the time as having said: '… the health of our seamen is invaluable, and to purchase that, no expense should be spared.'[8]

Nelson also directed Dr Snipe to visit Malta and to find a suitable location for a Naval Hospital and, on Snipe's recommendation, he urged the Admiralty to select the villa of a Count Bichi, which overlooked Grand Harbour, Valletta, as a suitable location; this later became the Royal Naval Hospital Bighi, Malta.

It is interesting to note that in 1804 Snipe ordered 30,000 gallons of lemon juice for the Mediterranean Fleet at one shilling a gallon. Sadly, it appears that Snipe, after visiting Messina in Sicily to obtain lemon juice, subsequently died having contracted an infection there. Nelson was impressed enough with the professionalism of Snipe that he wrote to the Admiralty requesting a pension for Snipe's widow, and stated in that letter:

> … I should testify to your Lordship His Character which I have much pleasure in doing for a better man in Private life nor a more able Man in His Profession I never met with and I much fear that his death was principally owing to his going to Messina for the purpose of buying lemon juice for the Fleet at home…[9]

Dr Thomas Trotter (1760–1832)

Thomas Trotter was another eminent Scottish physician and prolific author. He was born in Melrose and studied as a surgeon in Edinburgh. He joined the Royal Navy as a surgeon's mate in 1779 but was discharged at the end of the then wars against France, Spain and The Netherlands. Out of work, he joined a slaving ship and subsequently became an ardent anti-slaver. He returned to Edinburgh and qualified MD in 1788, and re-joined the Navy in 1790. He served on several ships under different admirals but was injured and invalided out of the service.

8 Nicholas Harris, *The Dispatches and Letters of Vice Admiral Lord Viscount Nelson*. Aug 1803 vii p.ccxv

9 Jane Bowden-Dan, 'Diet, dirt and discipline: Medical Developments in Nelson's Navy. Dr John Snipe's Contribution' in *The Mariner s Mirror* 90;3 (London: 2013), pp.260–272

Trotter was a leading medical reformer in the Royal Navy, publishing *A Review of the Medical Department of the British Navy, with a Method of Reform proposed* in 1790. His most famous publication was *Medicina Nautica: An essay on the Diseases of Seamen* (1797). Other subjects included publications on scurvy, drunkenness and, later, coal mines.[10]

Dr William Burnett (1779–1861)
William, later Sir William, Burnett was an eminent Scottish physician. He was born in Montrose, Scotland, and studied medicine at the University of Edinburgh. He served as an assistant surgeon under Sir John Jervis and was present at the Battle of Cape Saint Vincent. He also served at the Battle of the Nile and the Battle of Trafalgar. Burnett was then appointed to be in charge of prisoners of war at Portsmouth and in 1810 was promoted Physician and Inspector of Hospitals to the Mediterranean Fleet. He later became Inspector General of Naval Hospitals and Fleets and was then appointed as Director General of the Medical Department of the Navy, the first naval surgeon to hold this office. Arguably his most important innovation was the introduction of *Statistical Reports on the Health of the Navy* in 1840. On retirement, he became civil physician to the Navy and Physician in Ordinary to King William IV. He was made Knight Commander of the Bath and Knight Commander of the Royal Guelphic Order, a Hanoverian order of chivalry.

Five lesser-known Scottish trained naval surgeons

Sir William Beatty (1773–1842)
William, later Sir William, Beatty is believed to have studied at the University of Glasgow. In 1791, at the age of 18, he was examined by The London Company of Surgeons and qualified as a surgeon in the Royal Navy. He is best known for having cared for Admiral Lord Nelson at the time of his death aboard HMS *Victory* at the Battle of Trafalgar. After achieving fame at Trafalgar, Beatty studied further at the University of Edinburgh and later at the University of St Andrews. He was appointed Physician in Charge at Greenwich Hospital in 1822 where he remained for the next 17 years. He was also appointed Physician Extraordinary to King George IV and later to King William IV. He has been included here among the exalted ranks of Scottish naval surgeons because of his undergraduate and graduate education in Scotland.

Sir William Rae (1786–1878)
William Rae was born and educated in Dumfries and graduated MD from the University of Edinburgh. He initially joined the East India Company but transferred

10 Brian Vale and Griffith Edwards, 'Physician to the Fleet: The Life and Times of Thomas Trotter, 1760–1832' in *Journal of the Royal Naval Medical Service*. 98(London: 2006) pp.1–235.

to the Royal Navy as Surgeon in 1805. He served under the frigate captain Sir Edward Pellew (later Lord Exmouth). He led a distinguished naval career finally becoming Inspector General of Hospitals and Fleets of the Royal Navy. He was knighted in 1858.

Sir John Richardson (1787–1865)
John Richardson graduated in medicine from the University of Edinburgh in 1807 and became a surgeon in the Royal Navy. He joined Captain (later Sir) John Franklin in the search for the northwest passage between 1819 and 1822. He later travelled extensively in the Arctic. Richardson was knighted by Queen Victoria in 1846.

Sir James Clark (1788–1870)
James Clark took an arts degree at Aberdeen University, but then changed to medicine and studied at the University of Edinburgh, qualifying in 1809. On joining the Royal Navy, he served at RNH *Haslar* in Gosport and then at sea. At the end of the Napoleonic Wars in 1815, Clark left the navy and took up practice as a civilian. He published extensively in the medical literature and was later appointed Physician in Ordinary to Queen Victoria, with whom he found great favour, as he did with Prince Albert.

Sir John Liddell (1794–1868)
Sir John Liddell was a later generation Scottish surgeon who was born in Dunblane. He qualified in medicine at the University of Edinburgh and served at the Battle of Navarino in 1827, following which, for his work before and during the battle, he became the first recipient of the Gilbert Blane medal. He became director of the Royal Naval Hospital Bighi in Malta in 1827; was elected a Fellow of the Royal Society and was knighted in 1848. He later became Medical Director General (Naval), succeeding Sir William Burnett.

Conclusion

There are many more Scottish surgeons and physicians, both among the more junior ranks and those who reached very high positions in Britain's Royal Navy. It bears repeating that Scottish surgeons among the lower ranks accounted for 45 percent of all lower rank surgeons; 42 percent of upper rank surgeons and 62 percent of surgeons and physicians in leadership ranks.[11] This was at a time when Scotland accounted for only 10 percent of the population of Great Britain. Later, in 1850, *The Lancet* even protested against the 'clannish' domination by Scottish surgeons in the Royal Naval medical services.[12]

11 Christopher Myers, 'The Demography of Royal Naval Surgeons: Some views on the Process of Prosopography' in *Journal of World-Historical Information*, 2–3 (Pittsburgh: 2014–2015), pp.43–53.

12 Quoted in: Christopher Myers, 'The Demography of Royal Naval Surgeons: Some views on the Process of Prosopography' in *Journal of World-Historical Information*, 2–3

The National Archives at Kew have made accessible more than 1,000 journals of Royal Navy medical officers. These include journals of surgeons and assistant surgeons who served on His and Her Majesty's ships, Hospitals, Naval Brigades, shore parties and on emigrant and convict ships in the period from 1793 to 1880. These records give a detailed and fascinating idea of what life was like on board Royal Navy ships in the era.[13]

Surgeon Vice Admiral Sir James Watt, one of this author's past senior colleagues and later Medical Director General (Naval), is quoted as having said in 2005, 'The huge success of the Royal Navy in the eighteenth and nineteenth centuries was due in no small measure to the Naval Medical Service and the noble surgeons who gave the best possible care at that time to their patients, the seamen of the Royal Navy.'[14] That is why Naval surgeons (a large proportion of whom were Scottish) were instrumental in winning the Revolutionary and Napoleonic Wars.

Bibliography

Books

Haycock, David B., Archer, Sally, *Health & Medicine at Sea 1700–1900* (Woodbridge: Boydell Press, 2009)

McLean, David, *Surgeons of the Fleet* (London: Tauris, 2010)

Journal Articles

Bowden-Dan, Jane. 'Diet, Dirt and Discipline: Medical developments in Nelson's Navy. Dr John Snipe's Contribution' in *The Mariner s Mirror* 90.3 (London: 2013), pp.260–272

Caputo, S., 'Scotland, Scottishness, British Integration and the Royal Navy, 1793 to 1815' in *The Scottish Historical Review*, 97.1 (Edinburgh: 2018), pp.85–118

Chan, C. and Demetriades, A., 'The Contributions of James Carmichael Smyth, Archibald Menzies and Robert Jackson to the Treatment of Typhus in Royal Naval Vessels in the Late 18th Century' in *Journal of Medical Biography,* 31, 1 (London: 2023) pp.4–9

Myers, Christopher H., 'The Demography of Royal Naval Surgeons: Some views on the Process of Prosopography' in *Journal of World-Historical Information,* 2–3 (Pittsburgh: 2015), pp.43–53

Penn-Barwell, J. G., 'Sir Gilbert Blane FRS: the man and his legacy' in *Journal of the Royal Naval Medical Service*, 102 (London: 2016), pp.61–66

(Pittsburgh: 2014–2015), pp.43–53.

13 National Archive, 'Surgeons at Sea' https://cdn.nationalarchives.gov.uk/documents/surgeons-at-sea-highlights-guide.pdf. Accessed 14 April 2024

14 James Watt, 'Surgery at Trafalgar' in *The Mariner's Mirror,* 91:2 (London: 2005), pp.266–283.

Vale, Brian and Edwards, Griffith., 'Physician to the Fleet: The Life and Times of Thomas Trotter, 1760–1832' in *Journal of the Royal Naval Medical Service*. 98 (London: 2006) pp.1–235
Watt, James, 'Some Forgotten Contributions of Naval Surgeons' in *Journal of the Royal Society of Medicine*. 78, 9 (London: 1985), pp.753–762
Watt, James, 'Surgery at Trafalgar' in *The Mariner's Mirror*, 91, 2 (London: 2005), pp.266–283

Websites

National Archives, 'Surgeons at Sea' https://cdn.nationalarchives.gov.uk/documents/surgeons-at-sea-highlights-guide.pdf.
Wikipedia: 'The Gilbert Blane Medal':
https://en.wikipedia.org/wiki/Gilbert_Blane#The_Gilbert_Blane_Medal, accessed 23 November 2023.

5

A Forgotten Scottish Military Physician: Robert Henderson of Brighton (? –1808)

Max Cooper

Introduction

The contribution of Scottish doctors to the British military services over the past three centuries cannot be overstated. Many individuals considered in this book need no introduction. By contrast, the lives of other Scottish doctors remain unstudied or lost to history. One such 'forgotten' Scottish physician is Robert Henderson MD (Aberdeen, 1786) who became Physician to the Forces based in Brighton on the south coast of England in 1795. This Chapter presents glimpses into the life and world of Henderson, expanding upon a previously published biography.[1]

Scotland (before *c.* 1786)

Nothing is known about Henderson's life in Scotland beyond what is recorded in Munk's Roll of the Royal College of Physicians of London. This simply states that Henderson was:

> A native of Scotland, and a doctor of medicine of [Marischal College] Aberdeen, of 20 May 1786; was admitted a Licentiate of the College of Physicians 23 December 1793. He held the appointment of physician to the forces, and died at Brighton on 3 April 1808.[2]

1 Max Cooper, Menaka Jegatheesan, Carl Fernandes and Ben Whiston, 'Robert Henderson: Scottish doctor who was appointed Physician to the Forces (1795) and practised at Brighton, England' in *Journal of Medical Biography* (London: 2022). doi:10.1177/09677720221116550

2 William Munk. Robert Henderson. *Munk's Roll.* https://history.rcplondon.ac.uk/inspiring-physicians/robert-henderson (accessed 25 April 2024)

Even Henderson's year of birth remains unknown. It is of note that a Robert Henderson entered his 'first year of study' in medicine at Edinburgh University in 1783 and is recorded as an apprentice to the Royal College of Surgeons of Edinburgh in the same year.[3] Unfortunately, it is not possible to confirm whether this is the same individual, Henderson being such a common surname in Scotland.

Move to Brighton (*c.* 1786)

Henderson arrived in Brighton in about 1786. During the second half of the eighteenth century Brighton (then known as Brighthelmston) grew from a remote fishing village into a popular small town. It is unclear whether Brighton was Henderson's primary destination upon leaving Scotland. Indeed, he may have spent time in London considering openings for employment. Reasons for choosing Brighton are uncertain but probably lie in opportunities arising from the town's expanding population, association with the nobility and its reputation as a health resort for water therapy. Henderson's arrival in Brighton predates the ascent of Napoleon and thus his primary motive is unlikely to lie in future opportunities for advancement in the military services. Instead, Henderson may have chosen Brighton through Scottish acquaintances and three doctors are possible candidates. One is Thomas Blair (1764 –1853, of whom more later) who was born in Scotland, studied at Edinburgh and practised in Lewes. Another is the Scottish physician John Hunter (d. 1809) who was later noted at Brighton in the social company of Henderson.[4] Third – and the key contender – was Sir Lucas Pepys (1742–1830). Born in London, Pepys was the grandson of Dr Richard Russell FRS (1687–1759) who studied at Leiden and established Brighton as a popular resort for seawater therapy.[5] In 1772 Pepys married Jane Elizabeth Leslie, 12th Countess of Rothes (1750–1810). Through his Scottish wife, Pepys may have formed part of a network of doctors in London and Brighton associated with Scotland. Munk notes that in the late eighteenth century, Pepys practised in Brighton for the summer season. It is possible that by the mid–1780s he may have been keen to reduce his commitment there in order to pursue advancement within the Royal College of Physicians of London and in the Army Medical Services.

3 'Historical alumni: students of medicine 1762–1826, University of Edinburgh, https://collections.ed.ac.uk/alumni/record/77693?highlight=henderson (accessed 2 May 2024)

4 Max Cooper, Menaka Jegatheesan, Carl Fernandes and Ben Whiston. 'Disciples of Aesclepius': Glimpses into lives of the 'Gentlemen of the Faculty' of medicine in Brighton, England 1800–1809. Journal of Medical Biography. 2022. DOI:10.1177/09677720221131946

5 William Munk, Sir Lucas Pepys. *Munk's Roll.* https://history.rcplondon.ac.uk/inspiring-physicians/sir-lucas-pepys (accessed 25 April 2024).

Parish Doctor in Brighton (1794)

Early directories of Brighton show that Henderson offered private medical services in Brighton. The evidence also indicates that he worked as a parish doctor, perhaps until even as late as 1807.[6] His parish role is supported by the following account from December 1792:

> At a meeting of the Churchwardens and Overseers, held at the Castle Tavern, on 5 December that year, it was:- Ordered that Phœbe, the wife of William Hassell, be paid three guineas to get their bed and netts, which they had pledged to pay Dr Henderson for medicine.[7]

Henderson's service to the people of Brighton is evident in various accounts of a silver cup presented to him upon his departure for the nearby county town of Lewes. Among these descriptions, the following is the most informative:

> So truly are the Inhabitants of Brighthelmston of the distinguished attention which Dr HENDERSON evinced to the poor of that town, during the late general inoculation there, which, added to his medical skill, saved the lives of many, that they have presented him with a silver cup, as a small testimony of their gratitude with the following inscription engraven thereon:
>
> THE GENTLEMEN OF BRIGHTHELMSTON PRESENT THIS CUP TO DR HENDERSON, IN GRATEFUL ACKNOWLEDGEMENT FOR HIS ATTENTION TO THE POOR.[8]

In the early 1790s Henderson and his wife had three children in Brighton. The parish records are recorded:

Table 5.1 Henderson's children recorded in the parish records of St Nicholas' church, Brighton

Date	Parish Record
18 November 1792	burial record: 'Henderson Sophia d. [daughter] of Dr. Robert Henderson and his wife.'
30 January 1794	baptism record: 'HENDERSON Sophia Janet d. [daughter] of Robert M.D. and Sophia.'
22 May 1798	baptism record: 'HENDERSON John Hardinge (b.1.9.96) s. [son] of Robert M.D. and Sophia Elizabeth.'

6 Cooper et al., Robert Henderson,
7 J. A. Erredge, *History of Brighthelmston or, Brighton as I View it and others Knew it, with a chronological table of local events* (Brighton: E. Lewis, 1862), p.239.
8 Anonymous, *The Sussex Weekly Advertiser.* 14th April 1794, p.3.

Application for The 'Aesculapian Seat' in Lewes (1794)

Henderson is noted in March 1794 as offering his medical services in Lewes upon the departure of its regular physician:

> Dr ROBERTS, Having quitted Lewes, Dr HENDERSON, Licentiate of the Royal College of Physicians, in London, who has been settled for eight years past at Brighthelmston, begs leave to inform the inhabitants of Lewes, that he will attend (when sent for) upon the same footing that he attends the inhabitants of Brighton, and without making any charge for his journey.
>
> The Gentlemen of the country round are requested to send to Mr. W. Lee, Printer, who will immediately dispatch a messenger to Brighton for the Doctor.[9]

Soon after it became clear that his intention was to take up residence in Lewes:

> Dr Henderson, of Brighton, is about to take a house here, as successor to Dr Roberts[10]

This plan was evidently motivated by the vacancy in Lewes created by the departure of Dr Roberts. Nevertheless, a further factor may have made Lewes attractive: its location eight miles inland from Brighton. This may have been attractive in order for Henderson to distance his family from the threat of invasion by the French. William and Arthur Lee, the editors of the *Sussex Weekly Advertiser*, sometimes wrote in a witty style and termed the vacancy for a physician in Lewes as 'the Aesculapian seat in this town.'[11] Aesclepius was the Greco-Roman God of medicine whose rod took the form of a snake entwined around a staff.

One reference suggests that in March 1794 Henderson's move and appointment were now less certain. This appears to be because other physicians had entered the race:

> For the *Aesculapian* seat in this town, become vacant by the resignation of Dr Roberts, there are no less than three candidates, namely Dr Henderson, Doctor Blair and Doctor Remmington [*sic*][12]

Association with Dr Thomas Blair

The identity of Dr Roberts of Lewes and Dr Remington are unknown. By contrast, the biography of Dr Thomas Blair (1764–1853) is given in *Munk's Roll* of the Royal College of Physicians of London:

9 Anonymous, *The Sussex Weekly Advertiser*, 10th March 1794, p3
10 Anonymous, *The Sussex Weekly Advertiser*, 17th March 1794, p.3
11 Anonymous, *The Sussex Weekly Advertiser*, 24th March 1794, p.3
12 Anonymous, *The Sussex Weekly Advertiser*, 24th March 1794, p.3

> Thomas Blair [MD Edinburgh (1792) LRCP (1794)] was born in Scotland, and educated at Edinburgh, where he took his degree of doctor of medicine 12th September, 1792 (D.M.I. de Respiratione). He then repaired to Leiden for further improvement; returned to England, was admitted a Licentiate of the College of Physicians 25 June, 1794; and, settling at Lewes, practised there for several years. When the army returned after the Battle of Corunna, some detachments of the troops were quartered near Lewes, and among them typhus fever prevailed to a great extent. Dr Blair was appointed to the charge of these men, and for his skill and attention on this occasion he received the thanks of the Duke of York. In 1814 Dr Blair removed to Brighton, where he continued to practise with considerable repute until within a few years of his death, which occurred on 15 April, 1853, at the advanced age of 89. Dr Blair took an active part in the establishment of the Sussex county hospital, and was for many years one of its physicians.[13]

While Henderson undoubtedly visited Lewes and offered medical services to its residents, the evidence does not reveal with certainty whether or not he ultimately moved to the town. Indeed, it may be that the 'Aesculapian seat' in Lewes was awarded to Blair instead of Henderson. It is known that Blair practised in Lewes for many years and, therefore, perhaps Henderson was never appointed to the vacancy. An alternative explanation is that Henderson was indeed appointed and not Blair. This outcome is supported by Drew's record of the commissioned officers in the medical services of the British Army. Here it is stated that Thomas Blair may be the same individual who served as physician in the West Indies in 1795.[14]

Brighton's 'General Inoculation' Against Smallpox (1794)

Whatever the circumstances may have been, Henderson is recorded back in Brighton only a few months later partaking in a 'general inoculation'. Inoculation was the eighteenth century equivalent of 'vaccination' against smallpox through the application of small quantities of pustule fluid from patients with mild symptoms. Little appears to have been published about the 1794 general inoculation in Brighton. It was probably set in motion by the threat of the war with France and the need to protect the health of a significant military garrison already established in nearby Hove:

13 William Munk, 'Thomas Blair' in *Munk's Roll.* https://history.rcplondon.ac.uk/inspiring-physicians/thomas-blair (accessed 25 April 2024).

14 R. Drew, A. Peterkin and W. Johnston, *Commissioned Officers in the Medical services of the British Army 1660– 1960.* (Aberdeen: The University Press, 1925), p.89.

> In 1793, an encampment of about 10,000 troops, militia and regulars, took place at Hove, near this town, and continued, on account of some apprehensions of an invasion by the new Republic of France.[15]

Proposals for Brighton's 1794 'general inoculation' appear to have been contentious. Public fear over the risks of inoculation in vulnerable individuals and of inadvertently introducing smallpox can be inferred from a note in the *Scots Magazine* in January of the same year:

> The inhabitants of Brighton, at a vestry which was held there, decided against a general inoculation; of 5669, [amongst this number are] 1863 persons who never had the small-pox. Of the last [i.e. those who had never had smallpox], 26 were in a state of pregnancy.[16]

No numbers are recorded for Henderson's clinical outcomes during the general inoculation but overarching figures point to general success in Brighton. Nevertheless, published outcomes appear to justify public concern about inoculation, evident in increased mortality among children:

> The number of deaths occasioned by the general inoculation at Brighton, are now calculated at 25, principally children. About 2,000 submitted to the operation.[17]

Henderson's 'Great House' on West Street, Brighton

Henderson lived and undoubtedly practised from his 'great house' on West Street, Brighton. The location is not far from St Ann's Well, then an important source of chalybeate (mineral) water used for treating patients. West Street is of historical note for its association with the *King's Head Inn* where Charles II stayed on the night before his flight to France in 1659. No buildings from the original West Street remain today but it is possible to deduce where Henderson's house once stood (see photograph). Newspaper advertisements indicate that Henderson probably left this spacious residence in 1802, see below, but the reason for his departure is not recorded. Given his ongoing appointment to the British Army, this decision is unlikely to have been due to personal ill health.

> For Sale or To Let –
> On a Long Lease,

15 Erredge, *History of Brighthelmston*, p.169

16 Anonymous, *The Scots Magazine, Or, General Repository of Literature, History, and Politics* (Edinburgh: Alex Chapman and Company, 1794), p.49.

17 Anonymous, *The Sussex Weekly Advertiser*, 3rd March 1794, p.3.

> A Large Well-built Family House, situated about the middle of West-street, Brighton; Containing two sitting rooms; one drawing room, 20 feet square; six bed rooms; three garrets; kitchen; two cellars; wash-house; scullery; coal-house; two garden conveniences, and garden.
> For particulars, enquire of Dr Henderson, on the premises'[18]

Matters appear to have moved slowly. Similar advertisements almost one year later suggest that Henderson had decided to sell the house rather than to seek a 'long lease':

> to be SOLD by AUCTION,
> by Mr. H. R. ATTREE
> On Monday February 21, and following day,
> ALL the neat and genuine HOUSHOLD [*sic*] FURNITURE, China, and Glass, of DOCTOR HENDERSON'S great house, in West Street, Brighton.
> Also, from 15 to 20 dozen of Old Port Wine; and small quantity of Perry and Cyder.

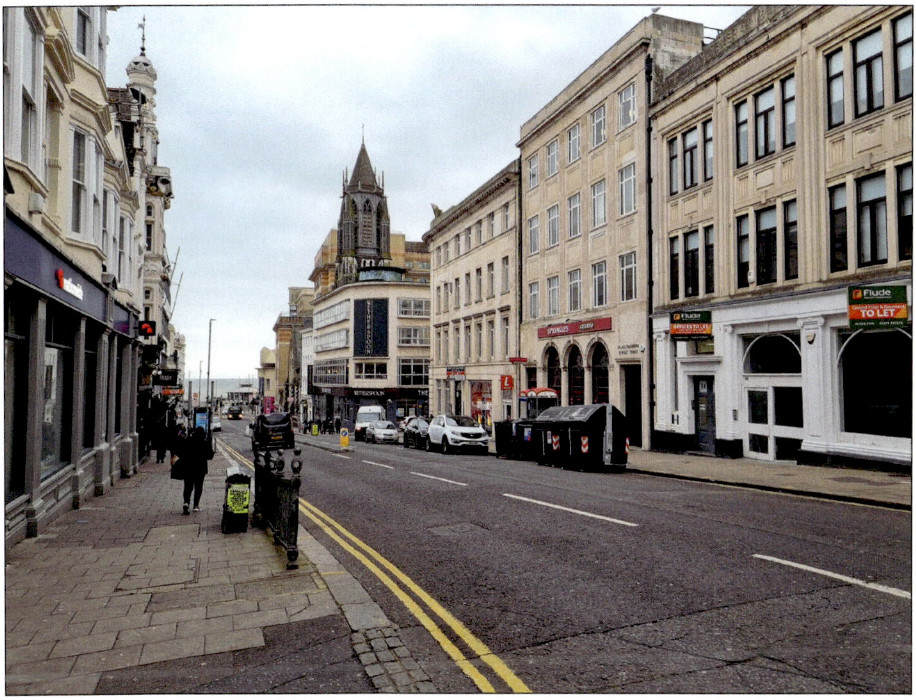

The central portion of West Street, Brighton, and approximate location of Henderson's 'great house'. This view looks south towards the sea. Photograph taken by M. J. F. Cooper in January 2024.

18 *The Sussex Weekly Advertiser,* 29th March 1802, p.3

> Catalogues to be had previous to the Sale, of Mr. H. R. Attree, at his Agency-Office, Brighton.[19]

Sir Lucas Pepys and Henderson's Appointment as a Garrison Physician (1795–1805)

As stated earlier, it is likely that in Brighton or London, Henderson met Sir Lucas Pepys who was well connected in medical, military and social circles. In 1794 Pepys was appointed Physician General to the army and, thus, to the Army Medical Board. Munk suggests that Pepys handpicked civilian physicians for the army. It is almost certain that Henderson's appointment constitutes an instance of this process. Munk leaves the following, somewhat barbed, description of Pepys:

> Sir Lucas made his appointments, we are told by Sir James McGrigor, from the ranks of civil life, without regard to previous service in the army, and proceeding on the principle that the army physician should possess the most extensive acquirements and the most complete education, he made it a rule that all candidates for appointment should be fellows or licentiates of the College of Physicians of London, of which body he was himself, during many of the years he was at the head of the Army Board, the president.[20]

Henderson was appointed Physician to the Forces on 6 October 1795. In his records of the commissioned officers in the medical services of the British Army, Drew gives the following records for Henderson's service:

> 1786: MD Marischal College Aberdeen; 5 October 1795: Physician to the Forces; 25 April 1798: half pay; 25 June 1802: half pay; 25 July 1803: full pay; 25 March 1805: half pay; 3 April 1808: died at Brighton. [21]

The dates of Henderson's return to full pay tally with periods of heightened threat of invasion by the French: 1795–8 and 1803–5. There is no evidence that Henderson saw action with the army and his role was, therefore, purely that of garrison physician.[22]

19 *The Sussex Weekly Advertiser*, 7th February 1803, p.3; *The Sussex Weekly Advertiser*, 21st February 1803, p.1
20 Munk, Sir Lucas Pepys, online op. cit.
21 Drew, Robert Henderson, p 93.
22 Cooper et al., Robert Henderson.

Investigating Brighton's Chalybeate Water

Henderson is noted as an advocate of local chalybeate (i.e. mineral spring) water and undertook basic experiments into its chemical properties. Erredge offers the following quotation about the chalybeate and these appears to constitute the only surviving words from Henderson's pen:

> This water, when first taken from the spring in a glass, in appearance greatly resembles a solution of emetic tartar in common water. The taste is not unpleasant, something like that upon a knife after it has been used in cutting lemons. It does not seem to contain the smallest portion of sulphur; it neither changes vegetable blues [*sic*], red, nor does it effervesce with alkaline salts, calcareous earths, magnesia, nor fossil alkali; neither does it change vegetable blues, green, nor does it effervesce with acids; yet it curdles soap, and renders a solution of it in various spirits milky.
>
> It seems to contain a considerable portion of calcareous earth, mixed with vitriolic acid in the form of its selenites, and also a considerable portion of iron, as will appear from the following experiment: Sixty-four ounces of this water by measure being evaporated to dryness, there was a residuum of a brownish colour, full of spiculæ, weighing eight grains, four ounces of which, with an equal quantity of charcoal, was made into a paste with oil, and calcined. On trying the calcined matter with the magnet, two pieces nearly in the metallic form adhered to it; and when put upon paper, at the distance of half an inch, moved in every direction with the magnet. These two pieces weighed one-eighth of a grain.
>
> The gross residuum neither effervesces with alkali nor acids, and is sufficiently soluble in water. This water becomes instantly transparent, like distilled water, on the addition of any of the mineral acids, especially the vitriolic. A solution of galls in common water, added to an equal portion of this water, becomes black like ink, in a few minutes.
>
> The chalybeate has been found serviceable in several cases of general debility, crapulas [a sense of intoxication resulting from excessive food or drink], indigestion, atony of the stomach, and fluor albus; and in all those diseases where chalybeate and tonic remedies are required, it promises, under due regulation, to be useful.[23]

23 Erredge, *History of Brighthelmston*, p.239.

Death and Descendants

Henderson was buried in his family vault at St Nicholas' church, Brighton, on 9 April 1808.[24] Newspaper records reveal Henderson's suffering and forbearance at his passing. It is suggested that this quality was rooted in his Christian faith:

> [Died]
> Yesterday, at his house in this town, R Henderson, Esq. M.D. after a very long and painful illness, which he supported with the firmness of a philosopher, and the resignation of a good Christian.[25]

Little is known about Henderson's descendants. It remains unclear whether he is the same Robert Henderson whose name is recorded on the monument of a Sophia Elizabeth Henderson (d. 1838) in the crypt of St Saviour's church, Bath.[26] In 1830 Henderson's daughter Sophia Janet married Captain William John Thompson Hood, who had served at the Battle of Trafalgar aboard HMS *Achille* aged 11.[27]

Conclusion

Henderson settled in Brighton around the time of his 1786 Doctor of Medicine degree from Aberdeen. Nothing is known about his origins in Scotland. In Brighton he worked as a parish doctor and practised privately. His receipt of an inscribed silver cup offers evidence of service to the poor. Although he did not see military action, Henderson's career was shaped by conflict with France. In 1794 he partook in Brighton's general inoculation and in 1795 was appointed Physician to the Forces in the capacity of a garrison doctor. The thread that runs through Henderson's career to connect the professional worlds of Brighton's medical faculty, London's Royal College of Physicians and the British Army medical services is likely to be Sir Lucas Pepys.

Henderson lived and practised in West Street, Brighton. Little is known about his treatments beyond the use of chalybeate water. Henderson possessed an analytical mind, leading him to examine the chemical composition of chalybeate water.

The evidence presented here brings together glimpses into Henderson's world: a silver cup for his medical skill, treating patients with chalybeate water, his 'great house' with scullery and garden conveniences, a surplus of port wine, perry and cider, his bereavement as a parent and stoical suffering when close to death. No image or tombstone of Henderson has come to light. It is not known whether any descendants exist. In his day, Henderson was an eminent figure in Brighton society. Beyond the

24 Anon, *The Sussex Weekly Advertiser,* 11th March 1808, p.3
25 Anon, *The Sussex Weekly Advertiser*, 4th April 1808
26 Cooper et al., Robert Henderson,
27 Cooper et al., Robert Henderson,

research presented here, he is sadly forgotten today. This Chapter stands as a monument to Robert Henderson MD and as a reminder of other forgotten Scottish military doctors who practised in England or served beyond the seas.

Acknowledgements

The author wishes to acknowledge the contributions of his colleagues and good friends who worked on a previous paper about Robert Henderson: Menaka Jegatheesan, Carl Fernandes and Ben Whiston. He would also like to thank Margaret Cooper and Sarah Cooper for reading drafts of this Chapter. Finally, thanks go to David Packham for his index of newspaper entries which proved invaluable for turning up some sources above.

Bibliography

Primary Sources

Sussex Weekly Advertiser (microfiche archive), the Keep archive, Falmer, Brighton

Books

Chapman, A., *The Scots Magazine, Or, General Repository of Literature, History, and Politics* (Edinburgh: Alex Chapman and Company,1794)

Drew, R., Peterkin, A. and Johnston, W., *Commissioned officers in the Medical Services of the British Army 1660– 1960* (Aberdeen: The University Press, 1925)

Erredge, J. A., History *of Brighthelmston or, Brighton as I View it and Others Knew it, with a chronological table of local events* (Brighton: E. Lewis,1862)

Articles

Cooper, Max J, Fernandes, Carl and Whiston, Ben. "Disciples of Aesclepius': Glimpses into lives of the 'Gentlemen of the Faculty' of medicine in Brighton, England 1800–1809' in. *Journal of Medical Biography*, 2022 (London: 2022). DOI:10.1177/09677720221131946

Cooper, Max, Jegatheesan, Menaka, Fernandes, Carl and Whiston, Ben, 'Robert Henderson: Scottish Doctor who was Appointed Physician to the Forces (1795) and Practised at Brighton, England' in *Journal of Medical Biography*. 2022 (London: 2022). doi:10.1177/09677720221116550

Websites

Anonymous, The University of Edinburgh historical alumni: students of medicine 1762–1826, https://collections.ed.ac.uk/alumni

William Munk, *Munk's Roll of the Royal College of Physicians of London*, https://history.rcplondon.ac.uk/inspiring-physicians

6

Waterloo – After the Glory Medical Care Case Reports and Surgical Results Following the Waterloo Campaign

Mick Crumplin

While there is now a considerable amount of available data about early nineteenth century battle trauma and military surgery, less is known about the post combat care received in general hospitals. Following the Waterloo campaign (primarily the period 15 June to 19 June 1815), less severe casualties were evacuated to parts of the Kingdom of The Netherlands, France, the German states and Britain. More seriously wounded men were taken to local hospitals around the environs of the battle and many British, German and some French wounded were transported back north to Brussels and Antwerp. Prussian casualties were housed at Louvain, Namur and Liège, and some French wounded were hospitalised at Termonde.

The large number of casualties after the Waterloo Campaign

The most serious challenge for the medical staff and their patients was the sheer number of wounded. Over the four-day principal part of the campaign, three armies totalling around 355,000 men, fought in four principal areas south of Brussels with the result that there were about 102,000 casualties (killed, died of wounds, wounded and missing). Over the four days of 15 to 18 June, there were 60,000 to 65,000 wounded men who required surgical care. More than 30,000 Allied and French were wounded on 18 June[1] and they were cared for by less than 1,000 surgical staff available of all nations – 255 of whom were serving on the medical staff or in Wellington's British

1 M. K. H. Crumplin, *The Bloody Fields of Waterloo, Medical Support at Wellington's Greatest Battle* (Godmanchester: Ken Trotman Publishing, 2015) p.28.

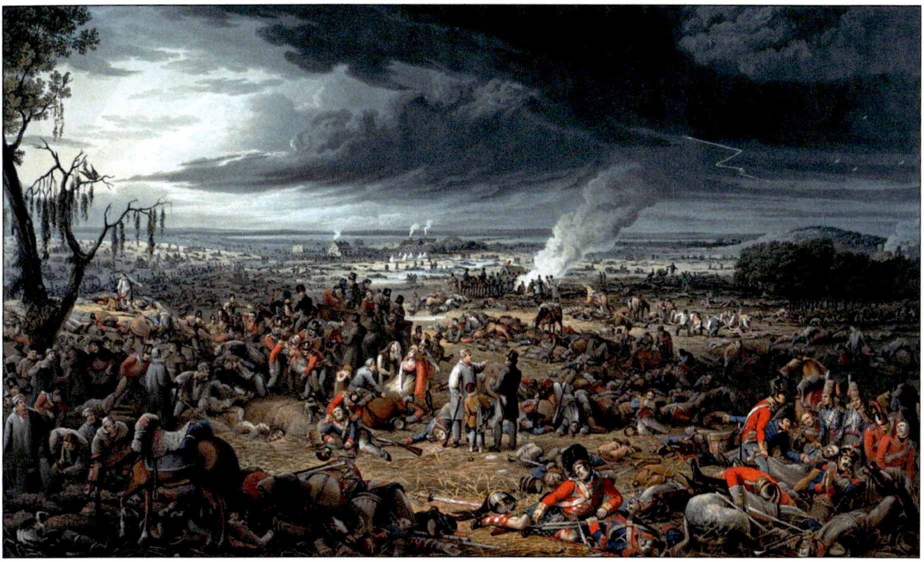

The dense masses of casualties after Waterloo preventing timely evacuation. Engraving by M. Dubourg after J. Heaviside Clark. (Author's collection)

and King's German Legion regiments.[2] There was little assistance from the *Service de Santé* since many of the French surgical staff had retreated, been wounded or been taken prisoner.

The crowding of the dead and wounded men and horses, as in many conflicts during these wars, was intense. The density of the casualties on the Waterloo fields was around 2,300 men (as well as hundreds of horses) per square mile of front, which is three times the density of that which occurred on the first day of the Battle of the Somme in 1916.[3] Thus, the removal of casualties from the combat areas took some time and many soldiers bled out or died of head and torso injuries before succour could reach them.

The British, Dutch-Belgian and German casualties found their way in to local cottages and hovels, but many crowded into the 1st Corps dressing station located at Mont St Jean where several thousand casualties were treated. The farm there was situated around 400 metres behind Wellington's ridge and front line.

The day after the battle, convoys of wagons and carts of all types trundled down from Brussels to collect the men who could not walk or ride and the slow painful journey north for the casualties began.

2 An estimate of 200–300 surgeons for each of the British/German, Dutch-Belgian, German, Prussian and fractured French field armies.

3 M. Crumplin and G. Glover, *Waterloo, After the Glory, Hospital Sketches and Reports on the Wounded after the Battle* (Warwick: Helion & Company, Warwick, 2019), pp.30–31.

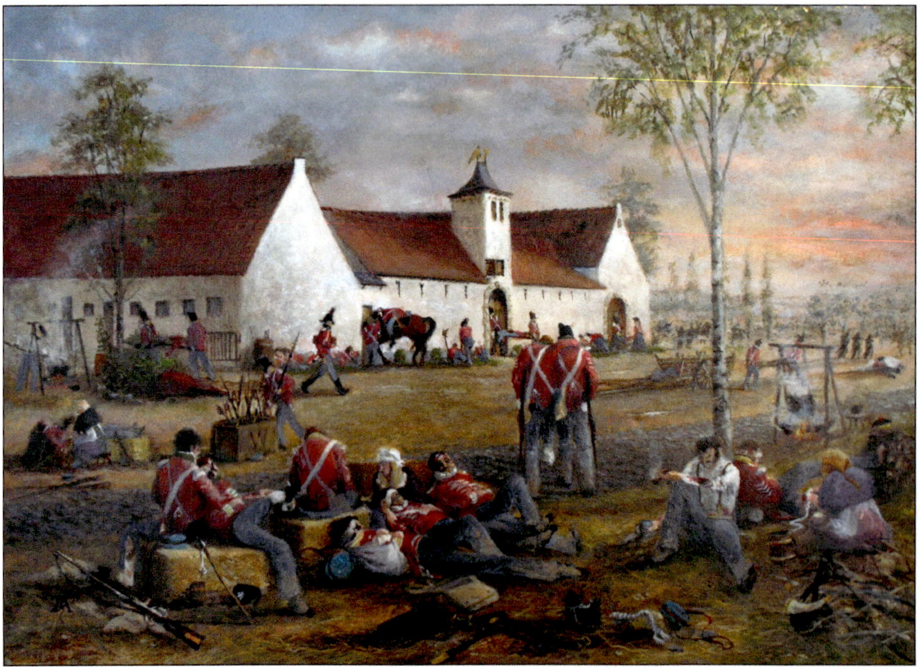

1st Corps field hospital at Mont St Jean, around 1800 hours 18 June 1815, oil painting by Beth Hough. (Author's collection)

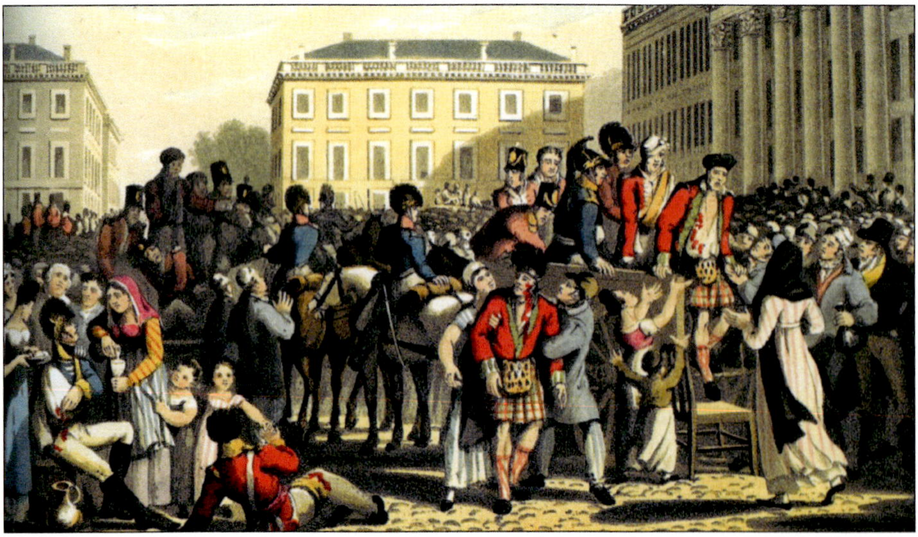

Wounded and civilians crowd Grande Place, Brussels. Engraving from page 19 of Walter Scott's *Poem*. (Author's collection)

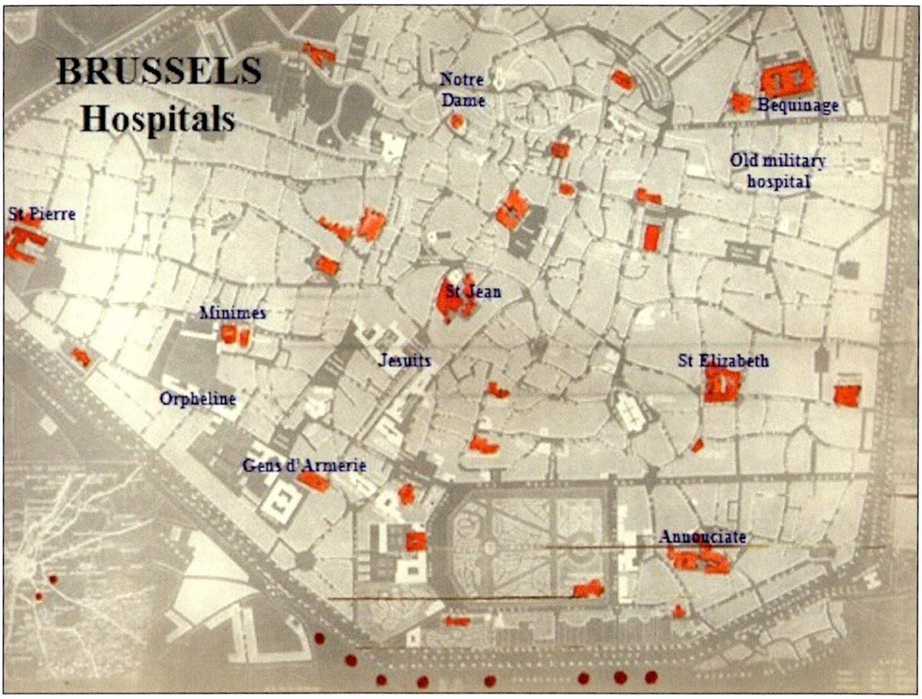

Siting of the five principal Allied hospitals (and others) in Brussels. (Author's collection)

It was not long before the city became packed with soldiers, the wounded, and civilians anxious to assist with the casualties. The cooperation of the citizens of Brussels was crucial to the care of the thousands of wounded, as was the assistance of many local medical staff, who included civilian doctors, students and retired professionals.[4]

The British Principal Medical Officer for the Waterloo Campaign was Inspector (later Sir) James Robert Grant (1771–1864), who had started as a surgeon's mate and graduated MD from King's College, Aberdeen. Grant was an experienced surgeon, who successfully liaised with the Dutch-Belgian authorities to accommodate the wounded in Brussels and Antwerp.

The hospitals caring for the Allied wounded

The main centres for the British, Dutch and German wounded were situated in Brussels and Antwerp, the latter acting as an overflow medical centre. The casualties were allocated to five principal hospitals; the Jesuit's, St Elisabeth, Annonciate,

4 Crumplin and Glover. *Waterloo, After the Glory*, p.43.

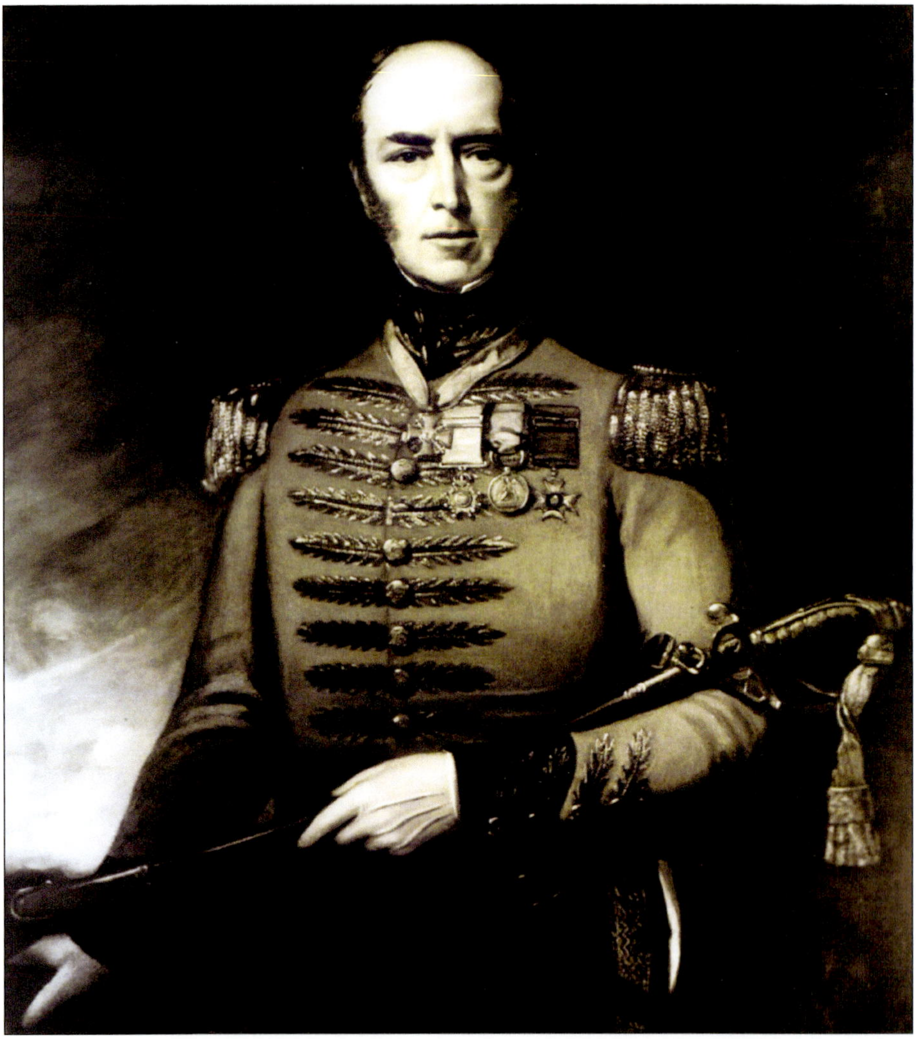

Inspector General Sir James Robert Grant. (Author's collection)

Minimes and the Gens d'Armerie, the latter accommodating some French patients. The five hospitals were collectively named *Le Grand Hôpital Général de l'Armée Alliée*. Each hospital had a senior medical member of staff in charge to supervise and assist with management and clinical challenges. Other Brussels medical facilities were the Orpheline, Notre Dame, Corderie (a rope factory where minor injuries were treated) together with the St Pierre and St Jean hospitals.

Antwerp hospitals included the Facon, another Corderie, St Elisabeth (the latter two for French patients), Augustine, Hotel du Nord and another Minimes. The principal

Prussian hospitals were at Louvain, Namur and Liège, with others in towns nearer the Rhine. Two Allied hospitals situated at the Channel ports of Ostend and Bruges were soon closed down to provide staff and equipment for the more inland units.

Grant worked closely and efficiently with Inspector General Sebald-Justinus Brugmans (1763–1819), an extremely capable Dutch physician who introduced careful measures to avoid seasonal contagion and succeeded in encouraging the citizens of Brussels to closely engage with the wounded in providing accommodation, bedding, bandages and food. Brugmans tried to avoid crowding of the casualties and, aside from small outbreaks of dysentery and fever, major epidemics in the crowded city during the warm weather conditions were prevented.[5] Many less experienced doctors, retired practitioners and others flocked to boost the medical forces in Brussels and Antwerp. It is perhaps important to emphasise that many Dutch and Belgian doctors had received their training in France or had been instructed by French military surgeons.

Professor John Thomson's analysis

Amongst the doctors who made the journey to Brussels from Britain, were two senior surgeons who had travelled from Scotland to assist and study the casualties of the Waterloo campaign. One of these was the principal investigator and author of the amassed medical data of the campaign. This was Professor John Thomson, Regius Professor of Military Surgery in Edinburgh (1765–1846) – he is considered in more detail in Chapter 8.

His companion was the most senior military surgeon of the Army Medical Department in Scotland, Deputy Inspector Dr William Somerville (1771–1860). These two surgeons visited hospitals in Brussels and Antwerp and subsequently wrote an account of the wounded with commentary. This was purely a critical qualitative analysis. Thomson did however, produce a useful collection of quantitative data in the form of case reports, hospital surgical outcomes, operations and wound types. In addition to these was a series of 176 primitive ink sketches giving, in most cases, detail of soldiers' names, units, the hospital in which they received care and their entry and exit wounds, often with a brief commentary. All of this data has allowed analysis of surgical results and clinical outcomes, both overall and from individual medical units.

Some of the patients were housed in the same billets they had occupied before the battles. Data was not available for the many wounded men cared for in private houses, and these numbered just over 4,100 patients. Each house containing casualties was marked by chalk inscriptions on the front door, indicating the number of patients and their nationalities. In Brussels there were 23 Dutch-Belgian surgical teams, 18 of which moved around the many billets, providing surgical advice and treatment.[6]

5 Crumplin and Glover, Waterloo, *After the Glory*, pp.56–70.
6 Crumplin and Glover, *Waterloo, After the Glory*, pp.61–62.

There is no readily complete data available concerning the management of the French casualties and the number of captured, wounded or dead French medical staff, as the *Armée du Nord* was fractured and retreating in many directions on its route back to France.

Allied and French Surgeons

As noted, the British Principal Medical Officer in Belgium was Inspector James Robert Grant, who probably remained in Brussels to supervise the care of the casualties. Dr John Hume (1782–1857) was the Duke of Wellington's personal physician and surgeon. From the southernmost part of the Kingdom of The Netherlands came Inspector General Sebald-Justinus Brugmans and the chief surgeon was François Kluyskens (1771–1843). Dutch surgeons present included Anthonius van Onsenoort (1782–1841), who remained in charge of the large hospital in Louvain, reserved for Prussian casualties and Karl Mergell (a German b. 1781) who was in charge of the surgical services for the Dutch-Belgian 1st Corps. A prominent Dutch surgeon and diarist of the Napoleonic war Louis Kerkhoves (or Kerkhoffs, 1789–1867), an experienced surgeon who had written of his participation in several previous campaigns. Surprisingly he does not seem to have helped with the wounded in the two cities (perhaps because he was suffering from 'burn out').

In the Prussian medical services, Director General Goercke (1750–1822) was the most senior medical officer in the Prussian medical service and the Superintendent of Military Hospitals was Karl von Gräfe (1787–1840). On the field, Blücher's local senior surgeon was Johann Voelzke (dates not found). The French Army during this campaign, had as its senior medical officer, Pierre François Percy (1754–1825), who was indisposed at the time and the Emperor's surgeon, who also looked after the Imperial Guard, was Dominique Jean Larrey (1766–1842).[7] Larrey, probably the most noted and revered surgeon of the era, was twice captured by the Prussians and almost executed.

Thomson's Case Reports and Surgical Data

Professor Thomson's carefully collated case reports, casualty and surgical data have been deposited in the Edinburgh University Library and examples of these are given below. Thomson was born in 1765 and, after a medical apprenticeship and then serving as house surgeon and studying anatomy in London under John Hunter, he was appointed surgeon to the Royal Infirmary of Edinburgh. In 1803, at the

7 E. Evrard, J. Mathieu, R. J. François, R. Moorthamers, *Esaculape aux Armeés, 500 ans de Médecine en Belgiques* (Brussels: Société Scientifique du Service Médical Militaire, 1997), pp.73–84.

advanced age of 38 years, he became a hospital mate, an appointment which would allow him to serve in a military hospital in the event of an invasion. Three years later he was appointed the Regius Chair of Military Surgery at the University of Edinburgh, and following Waterloo he was promoted to the rank of Staff Surgeon to the Forces. In 1832 he also held a Chair in General Pathology. He died in Edinburgh in 1846.

The first collection of papers consisted of 25 individual clinical case reports. The series continues with a series of simple, black, etched line drawings of wounds with brief descriptions, followed by a series of wound classifications, returns of the outcomes of surgical procedures and general mortality figures for the campaign. Clearly the cases that are enumerated in all the papers are of a more serious nature. The numbers are small in relation to the total number of wounds managed, since medium or minor injuries are not considered.

The handwritten clinical case reports are easily read and were compiled by six staff surgeons and three hospital assistants. The histories were taken from 18 British soldiers and seven French prisoners of war. Different anatomical regions were well represented. There were six head and neck injuries (one death), two chest wounds (one death), three abdominal or groin wounds (one death), six upper limb cases (four deaths) and eight hip or lower limb wounds (eight deaths). These figures give an overall 60 percent mortality rate. The small sample gives an impression of the challenges of bleeding and sepsis faced by the military surgical staff. The high-risk attending wounds of the thigh and hip are apparent and surgical results for this high-risk injury would only start to improve 100 years later.

Thomson's Sketches

John Thomson created 176 line drawings with 3 duplicates. Various nationalities were represented among the casualties, yet the numbers were clearly skewed towards the Allied force. There were 106 British or King's German Legion, 37 French, 14 German, 3 Dutch and 16 unspecified patients. Of the 98 British cases selected, 78 percent were serving in the infantry. Once again different anatomical areas were well represented among the injuries. There were 49 head or neck, 33 chest, 25 abdominal or pelvic, 14 back or buttock and 52 limb cases illustrated. The sketches are simple in construction and often labelled with the entry and/or exit wounds, and, as mentioned, many of the drawings give the soldiers' names and their units. The hospital is also recorded at the left top of many case sketches. Several French prisoners of war names are omitted.

Two examples of the sketches with the relevant contemporary notes are given below. The first case is that of Samuel Pritchard of the 4th (King's Own) Regiment who was wounded by a musket ball which passed through his forehead and became lodged behind the left eye. Sir Charles Bell produced a watercolour of this patient's head and was the only example of a matching process, tying Bell's Waterloo paintings together with Thomson's sketches.

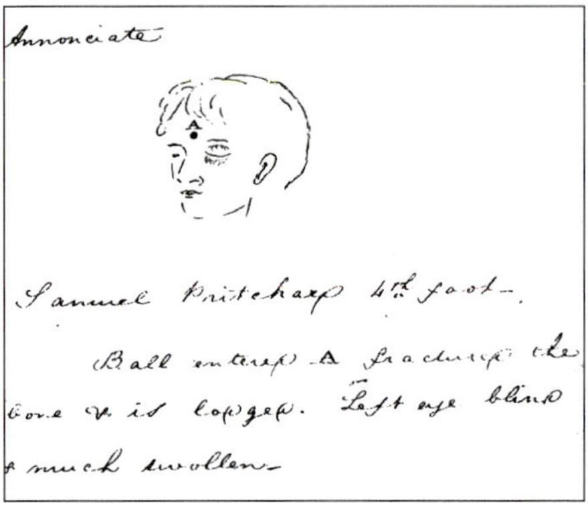

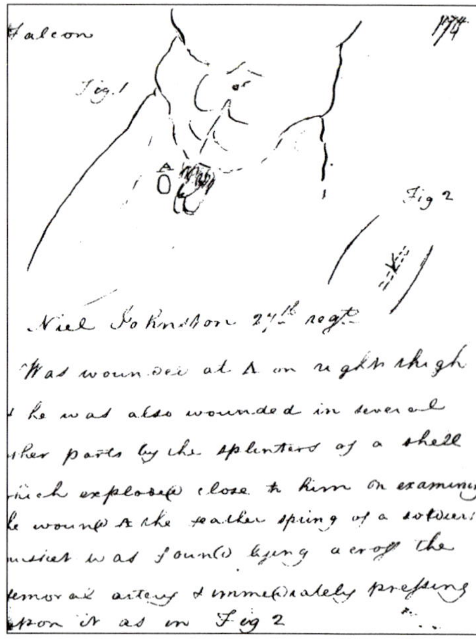

Above: Sketch and description of Private Samuel Pritchard's wound. (Reproduced courtesy of University of Edinburgh library)

Right: Private Niel Johnson's right groin wound. (Reproduced courtesy of University of Edinburgh library)

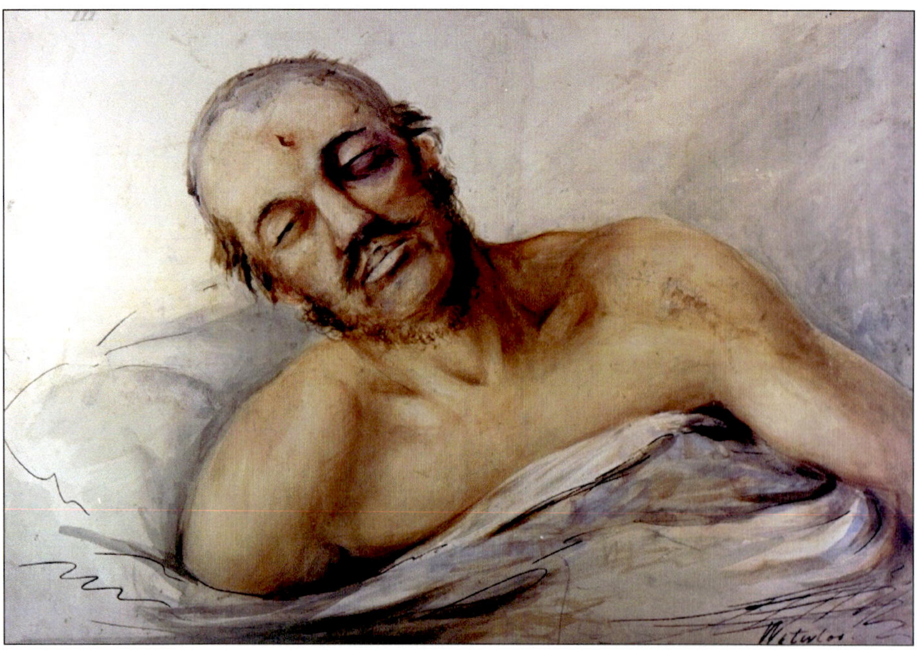

Private Samuel Pritchard. Watercolour by Charles Bell. (Reproduced courtesy of Museum of Military Medicine)

Bell was involved in Pritchard's treatment and remarked that he would have tried to remove the missile by approaching it via a lateral incision in the orbit.

Private Johnson of the 27th (Inniskilling) Regiment was struck by several splinters of shell casing. One wound occurred in the right groin. When this wound was explored it revealed the feather, spring (part of a musket's flintlock mechanism) of his or another man's musket which had been shattered, lying across the patient's femoral artery and compressing the vessel.

Analysis of Wounds Treated at the Jesuit's Hospital

The next collection of documents studied were those that gave data on wound types, clinical outcomes, surgical procedures and results. The first document of that group emanated from the large Jesuit's Hospital in Brussels. The paper is dated 16 July 1815 and the hospital was in the charge of the experienced Irish staff surgeon, John Hennen.

The next line consists of headings denoting the areas of the body injured; head, thorax, abdomen, upper then lower extremities. At right angles to these headings, are subheadings giving further detail or outcomes for each part wounded, such as, under 'thorax', 'one side', and 'both sides', under 'abdomen', 'cavity of' or 'pelvis' and for upper and lower extremities, there are classified the various parts of the limbs damaged. For each section of area wounded there then followed general outcome results – 'total' patients, 'convalescent' or 'died'. On the right side of this table, at right angles to the above categories are written, 'Gun shot wounds', 'Incised wounds',

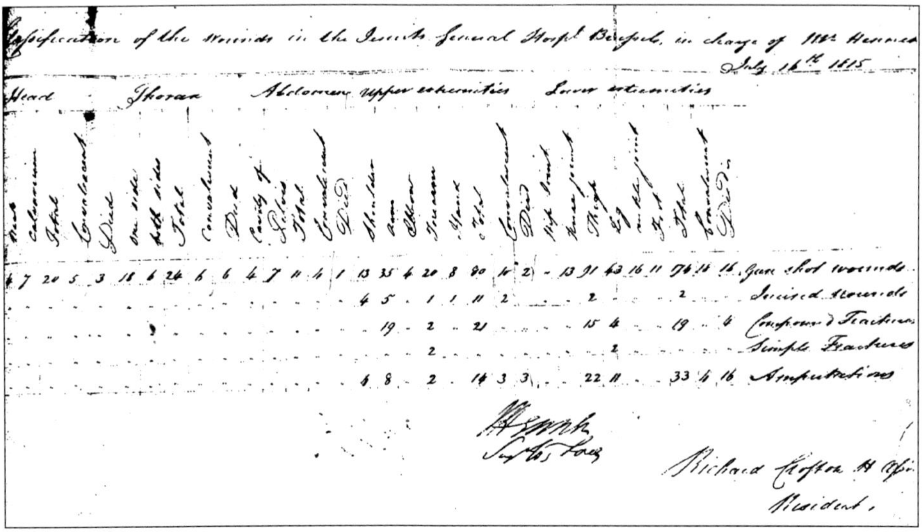
Classification of the Wounds in the Jesuits General Hospl Brussels, in charge of Mr Hennen
July 16th 1815
Head Thorax Abdomen Upper extremities Lower extremities
Gun shot wounds
Incised wounds
Compound Fractures
Simple Fractures
Amputations

Classification, causation and outcomes of various wounds recorded on 16 July 1815 at the Jesuit's Hospital Brussels. (Reproduced courtesy of University of Edinburgh library)

'Compound fractures', 'Simple fractures' and 'Amputations'. The document is signed by Staff Surgeon John Hennen and Hospital Assistant Richard Crofton (Resident).

We can from these data, study several aspects of survival under the pre-anaesthetic and pre-antiseptic conditions at these times. For example, if we select the fate of soldiers wounded in their lower limbs, extracting information from this table, we may note incidence, wound sites and mortality. Thus, in the Jesuit's Hospital there were 173 soldiers wounded in the thigh, leg and foot. This compares with 80 cases of men hurt in the upper limbs. Of the 173 patients, 91 had thigh injuries, 13 knee joint damage, 42 men were injured in the leg and 27 wounded in the ankle or foot. All but two injuries were from gunshot injury – the other two men were wounded by sword strikes. Of those categorised (clearly incompletely) in the table, only 19 were listed as 'compound' injuries, the other two listed were 'simple' fractures, where the bone had not been exposed to the air. Of the cases listed, 33 underwent amputation and 48 percent of these men died. Overall in this small analysis the mortality rate for lower limb injuries in this hospital was nine percent. Thus we may conclude that, in this hospital, lower limb injuries were twice as frequent as those in the upper limb and the high mortality rate for thigh fractures was likely due to delayed evacuation and treatment, sepsis and/or haemorrhage.

Outcomes of surgical operations

Although there were other hospital results set out in a non-standard tabular format, the final table reproduced here gives results solely for surgical operations which were carried out in the St Elisabeth Hospital in Brussels up until 1 August 1815, i.e. for two weeks or so after the Battle.

This survey of 134 patients undergoing surgery lists the surgical procedure or area operated on in the left column. Across the top, set at right angles, are recorded the categories; 'Operations', 'Recovered', 'Died', Under Treatment', 'Transferred' and 'Total'. Most of the cases are those soldiers undergoing limb surgery, but there are listed four head injuries and one carotid artery injury. There were 67 lower limb injuries, of which 41 were compound thigh wounds. Three of four head injuries died, but the man with the carotid artery wound lived. Of the 134 cases, 38 patients died (28 percent). This report is signed by Physician to the Forces, William Wray, who died in 1817.

From study of all Thomson's collected hospital reports it has been possible to extract the mortality rates for the various areas of the body injured. This composite series comprised 322 patients from the five Allied hospitals in Brussels. Before listing these, it is important to recall that to reach a general hospital alive after injury was a strong survival indicator in itself. Thus many head, torso and limb injuries would have resulted in a rapid demise from bleeding on the field, which helps explain the apparently low death rate for some of those categories given below. The mortalities in percentages by wound site were; head and neck 15, thorax 24, abdomen and pelvis nine, upper limb three and lower limb, nine percent.

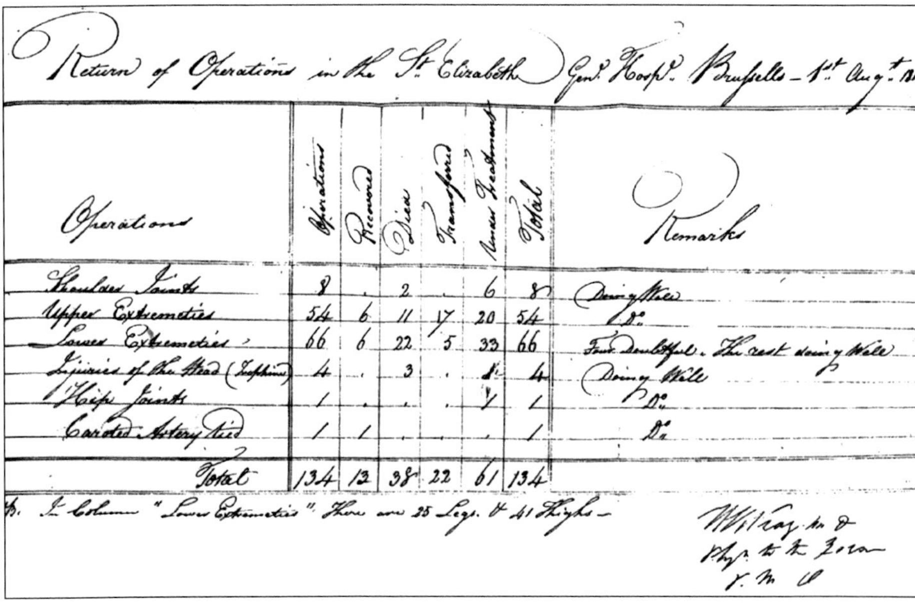

Return of Operations in the St Elizabeth Genl Hospl Brussells – 1st Augt 1815

Operations	Operations	Recovered	Died	Transferred	Under Treatment	Total	Remarks
Shoulder Joints	8	.	2	.	6	8	Doing Well
Upper Extremities	54	6	11	17	20	54	Do.
Lower Extremities	66	6	22	5	33	66	Four doubtful. The rest doing Well
Injuries of the Head (Trephine)	4	.	3	.	1	4	Doing Well
Hip Joints	1	.	.	.	1	1	Do.
Carotid Artery tied	1	1	.	.	.	1	Do.
Total	134	13	38	22	61	134	

N.B. In Column "Lower Extremities" There are 25 Legs & 41 Thighs –

[illegible]

Return of cases undergoing surgery at the St Elizabeth Hospital, Brussels.
(Reproduced courtesy of University of Edinburgh library)

The next issue addressed is the place and the timing of interventional surgery. A small number of documents report results from two hospitals with a combined total of 113 patients. These papers record 'primary' and 'secondary' operations in one paper and also surgery performed 'elsewhere' or later, in a 'general hospital' in the second paper. Both primary surgery and surgery carried out elsewhere infer earlier intervention – in other words somewhat sooner than in the general hospital setting. The mortality rates for primary surgery and surgery carried out elsewhere were 22 percent and 38 percent respectively, while surgery performed in the two general hospitals carried mortality rates of 37 and 55 percent respectively. This confirms (inevitably with some case selection) a survival advantage with early surgery carried out in the regimental or field hospital settings.

The Hospitals Compared

Following this is the need to address the returns and surgical results emanating from each of the five Allied general hospitals. Unfortunately, we do not know for each unit what proportion of the cases arrived early or later, or whether in some there were French prisoners treated later than the Allies. Neither can we surmise whether there were more or less capable surgeons or a higher proportion of badly injured men in each hospital. However, the results shown below in the table are of interest in their variation.

Surgical mortality in the five principal Allied hospitals in Brussels (for 348 patients)					
Hospital	Elizabeth	Jesuits	Annonciate	Gens d'Armerie	Minimes
Patients	134	103	51	25	35
percent mortality	28	28	37	56	40

The patient numbers in each hospital are in the upper row; the percent mortality is shown in lower row

There is a considerable discrepancy between the mortality rates and case allocation/ selection must have been a significant influence. It is notable that the two hospitals which had the most cases recorded had the lowest, and identical, death rates. It is interesting that the Gens d'Armerie hospital had smaller numbers yet the highest mortality, probably as a result of late presenting French surgical cases.

Overall, in regard to all the cases recorded in Thomson's report from Brussels, there was a series of 6,636 wounds treated in hospital patients of whom 745 died (an 11 percent mortality). Surgery was undertaken on 508 patients, and of these, 212 died (42 percent). So, the mortality almost quadrupled if surgical intervention took place. The mortality for Allied wounded in Belgium after Waterloo was 850 of 9,500 patients (nine percent), in keeping with Hodge's estimates for the war.[8]

French Casualties

Little has been said of French casualty figures. Data are incomplete as yet, but there was one small series of 259 wounded French prisoners of war recorded in Brussels. These were housed in the Gens d'Armerie Hospital under the care of Staff Surgeon Dr Theodore Gordon (1786–1836). He had arrived late to the scene, as had Charles Bell, who undertook several operations on these high-risk French casualties. Most of these cases were significantly immobilised by their injuries and could not have fled the battlefield. Also, having been collected late from the field, most were in a wretched state and not a few died before surgery could be carried out. Of the 259 patients, 146 (56 percent) had lower limb wounds (86 with compound femoral fractures). Of the 146 cases with hip, thigh or leg injuries, 32 underwent amputation (22 percent).[9] Mortality figures were not available.

8 W. B. Hodge, 'On the Mortality Arising from Military Operations' (London: paper read to the Statistical Society of London, 21 April 1856), p.223.

9 M. Crumplin and G. Glover, *Waterloo, After the Glory*, pp.105–106.

Surgical outcomes from the Waterloo Campaign

In the author's opinion, the surgical results and outcomes following the Waterloo campaign, likely fell short of the (admittedly limited) successes that had been achieved at the end of the Peninsular War of 1808 to 1814. The reasons for this are that the campaign in the Netherlands was hurriedly prosecuted and there were fewer British staff and regimental surgeons with Peninsular experience available. Nevertheless, the cooperation and harmony between the Dutch, German and British surgeons and a few physicians, went some way to compensate for these issues.

Modern legacies of the Waterloo Campaign

There remain today two recent legacies recalling the suffering and medical support after this iconic campaign. The first is a surgical display, a carefully exhibited collection of instruments, models, books, battlefield artefacts, paintings and a small panorama, highlighting the surgical services and the patients' challenges. This unique exhibition, labelled in three languages, is housed in the farm of Mont St Jean around 400 metres behind Wellington's front line. The farm was the principal field dressing station for Allied casualties on the day of Waterloo.

The other project is an ongoing charitable effort to bring together British and Foreign veterans who have suffered significant bodily or psychological trauma following combat and service in their armed forces. They form part of teams which include professional British and Belgian archaeologists, who supervise the veterans' work in digging around the farm and many other Waterloo campaign sites. The charity is named 'Waterloo Uncovered' and it has proved a remarkable success.[10] To enhance the display in the farm, the teams have uncovered battlefield artefacts, skeletal remains and surgically removed (bony) body parts, buried in medical waste pits at the eastern fringes of the farm.

Bibliography

Primary Sources

Thomson, J., *Report of Observations made in the British Military Hospitals in Belgium after the Battle of Waterloo, with some remarks on amputations* (Edinburgh: William Blackwood; London: T Cadell & W Davies, 1816)

Thomson, J., Somerville, W., *Collection of Sketches and Reports of Wounded at the Battle of Waterloo* (Edinburgh: Centre for Research Collections, Edinburgh University Library, Shelf Marks 594D & 595D, 1816)

10 https://waterloouncovered.com.

Secondary Sources

Crumplin, M. K. H., *The Bloody Fields of Waterloo, Medical Support at Wellington's Greatest Battle* (Godmanchester: Ken Trotman Publishing, 2015)

Crumplin, Michael and Glover, Gareth, *Waterloo, After the Glory, Hospital Sketches and Reports on the Wounded after the Battle* (Warwick: Helion & Company, 2019)

Evrard, E., Mathieu, J., François, R. J., Moorthamers R, *Esaculape aux Armeés, 500 ans de Médecine en Belgiques* (Brussels: Société Scientifique du Service Médical Militaire, 1997)

7

'The Picture is Distressing to Gaze Upon' – Charles Bell and the Expressions of War

Cat Irving

The soldiers returning to the south coast of England in January 1809 had been through difficult times. General Sir John Moore had taken control of a large military force in Spain two months earlier to help the Spanish drive the French out of Spain, backed by reinforcements under the command of General David Baird.[1] By Christmas 1808 they were forced into a 300 mile retreat to Corunna across mountain paths muddy with heavy rain that turned into sleet and snow, in clothes ill-suited to the bitterly cold weather conditions. There was little food, and even when food could be found, many of the mules that might have transported it had already died of exhaustion. Morale was low, and discipline began to break down; when they discovered a wine repository in the village of Bembibre, more than 1,000 men had to be left behind due to intoxication.[2] The sick and injured were left too. On reaching Corunna on the northwest coast of Spain, the depleted force defended the port, but at the cost of Moore's life – lost after taking round shot to his left shoulder. The survivors boarded ships back to England.

1 E. Niderost, 'Dismal British Retreat to Corunna' in *Warfare History Network* (April 2009) www.bing.com/search?pglt=43&q=nidersot+Dismal+British+Retreat+to+Corunna&cvid=95cf097fd2ec433e995613315042f171&gs_lcrp=EgZjaHJvbWUyBggAEEUYOdIBCDMxODhqMGoxqAIIsAIB&FORM=ANNTA1&PC=ASTS (accessed April 18, 2024)

2 Charles Oman, *A History of the Peninsula War*, (Oxford: Clarendon Press, 1902), p.566.

A Comminuted Fracture Among the Corunna Wounded at Portsmouth

Of the 28,000 men who returned from Spain at least 5,000 were sick or wounded.[3] Makeshift hospitals were set up in Portsmouth. A painting on display in Surgeons' Hall, Edinburgh shows one of the men who was treated there. He sits, torso uncovered, right arm resting on a pillow before him with an obvious wound on his upper arm.[4] The surgeon treating him describes the 'apparently trifling nature of the wound'[5] – though the key word here is 'apparently'. The diagnostic equipment used today was not available and so the surgeon's conclusions were reached by exploring the wound with a finger pushed into the defect in the bone – the wound was likely caused by a musket ball. The exploration revealed the jagged bone fragments of a comminuted fracture. This kind of shattered bone is not only difficult to heal well, but when open to the air, as was the case here, carries a high risk of infection. The doctors treating this man would not have had a modern understanding of germ theory, but they would be very familiar with the potentially fatal sepsis so frequently seen following injuries like this.

Today a comminuted fracture is usually treated surgically, using materials such as surgical screws, plates or wires to immobilise the fracture but these options were not yet available. Amputation replaced shattered limbs and torn flesh with a single, clean surgical wound, intended to increase the patient's chance of survival. There was, of course, no anaesthesia at the time for either investigation of the wound or for amputation of the limb. Pain relief would only come from either brandy or, if the patient was lucky, opium or laudanum. After this particular amputation, the surgeon macerated the bone of the amputated limb and wired the fragments together, to illustrate the effects of this kind of injury on the bone. Today that wired bone specimen is displayed next to the portrait of the soldier in Surgeons' Hall Museums.[6] There is no evidence as to who young man was, or what happened to him post-surgery. The doctor who treated him, however, was Charles Bell – later Sir Charles Bell.

Charles Bell (1774 – 1842)

Bell was born in Fountainbridge in Edinburgh in 1774, the youngest son of the Rev. William Bell, who died when Charles was five years old. His medical education began at the University of Edinburgh, but he was also apprenticed as a surgeon apothecary

3 Figures taken from M. K. H. Crumplin, and P. H. Starling, *A Surgical Artist at War: The Paintings of Sir Charles Bell 1809–1815* (Edinburgh: Royal College of Surgeons of Edinburgh, 2005).
4 Collection of the Royal College of Surgeons of Edinburgh, accession number GC.13830
5 Crumplin and Starling, *A Surgical Artist at War*, p.28.
6 Collection of the Royal College of Surgeons of Edinburgh, accession number GC.13830-1

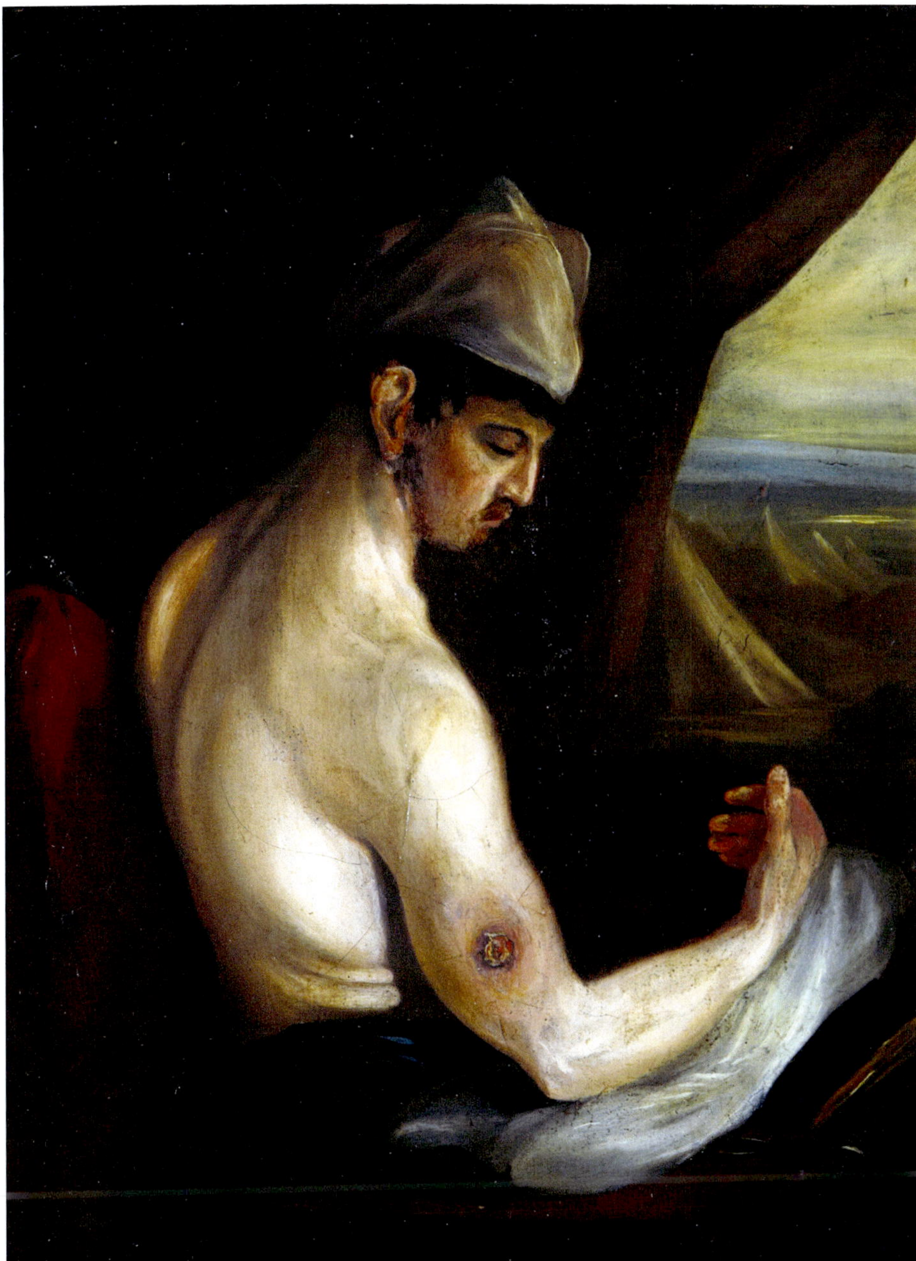

Gunshot wound to the humerus, by Charles Bell. (Reproduced courtesy of Surgeons' Hall Museums, Royal College of Surgeons of Edinburgh)

to his older brother John in 1792,[7] who also taught extramural anatomy classes, which Charles attended.

In 1804 aged 30, Charles Bell went to London, with 'a light purse, without almost a single acquaintance, and with very few introductions.'[8] Letters to his brother George show him actively courting the important medical men of the time. In his first week in the city he called on a number of influential individuals including Matthew Bailie, Maxwell Gartshore, John Abernethy, William Lynn and Leigh Thomas. Sir Astley Cooper invited him to dinner, and he met James Wilson, who ran the Anatomy School in Great Windmill Street set up by William Hunter.[9] This connection is important – Bell went on to buy the Great Windmill Street Anatomy School in 1812, with what constitutes 'all my money to the last penny' and 'eighteen pence more.'[10] Some of these men would become close friends. Bell dedicated the second edition of his *A System of Operative Surgery* to William Lynn.[11]

Charles Bell's Artistic Talent

Both John and Charles were talented artists – their mother Margaret Morice was a gifted artist who encouraged their abilities, and paid for regular lessons from the leading Scottish painter, David Allen. In 1809 Charles volunteered to treat the wounded returning from Corunna, fulfilling an ambition; in a letter to his brother George two years earlier, he had stated '...of all things I should like to be kept and sent to the armies as a surgeon.'[12] While in Portsmouth he used his artistic talents to make sketches that he later worked into a collection of oil paintings now held at Surgeons' Hall. Bell sold his collection to the Royal College of Surgeons in 1825 for £3,000 – equivalent to approximately £170,000 today. As well as the Corunna oils, the collection included anatomical and pathological preparations, and wax models that Bell had used for teaching. These waxes almost induce the stench of the dissection

7 The indenture document between John Bell, Surgeon Apothecary, and Charles Bell is held in the archive at the Royal College of Surgeons of Edinburgh, and can be viewed online at https://archiveandlibrary.rcsed.ac.uk/special-collections/incorporation-of-surgeons-and-barbers-of-edinburgh/apprenticeship-indentures-1653-1836/1230978-indenture-between-john-bell-surgeon-apothecary-in-edinburgh-and-charles-bell-his-brother-withrobert-bell-writer-to-the-signet-as-cautioner-1?

8 John Struthers, 'Sir Charles Bell' in *Historical Sketch of the Edinburgh Anatomical School* (Edinburgh: Maclachlan and Stewart,1867), pp.44–55.

9 *Letters of Sir Charles Bell selected from his correspondence with his brother George Joseph Bell* (London: John Murray, 1870), pp.20–1.

10 Struthers, "Charles Bell", p.48.

11 The second edition was published in 1814, and the dedication reads: '*To William Lynn, Esq. Surgeon of the Westminster Hospital, this volume is inscribed in testimony of friendship, by the Author*'. Charles Bell, *A System of Operative Surgery Founded on the Basis of Anatomy* (:London: Longman & Co.,1814).

12 Letter dated 21 May 1807 in *Letters of Sir Charles Bell*, p.96.

room, different to the sanitised wax anatomy models which had been produced in Italy throughout the previous century. He seems to have been following John, whose own anatomical illustration sought to recreate the real experience of working from cadavers. In *Engravings of the Bones, Muscles and Joints*, John Bell criticised such idealised representations, saying that anatomical illustration too often suffered from 'the capricious interference of the artist, whose rule it has too often been to make all beautiful and smooth, leaving no harshness.'[13]

Charles Bell's Corunna paintings are particularly interesting when considered in relation to a work he had begun in Scotland, but completed in London. *Essays on the Anatomy of Expression in Painting* was published in 1806, and republished in 1824 as *The Anatomy and Philosophy of Expression* with reflections on what he had observed as a war surgeon. It shows Bell's ambition; he was aware of his talents as both an anatomist and illustrator, and this publication almost seems a supplication to the Royal Academy.[14] William Hunter had been the Royal Academy's first Professor of Anatomy when it was founded in 1768. Hunter had been a patron of the arts and a collector, but did not have Bell's great artistic talent; the position of Professor of Anatomy at the RA seemed a perfect fit for Bell, who taught anatomy to artists including Edwin Landseer and David Wilkie.[15] It was not a position he would hold, however. In spite of the success of his book, which was valuable from both an artistic and medical perspective, when the position became vacant in 1808 it would go to Anthony Carlisle.[16]

The central tenet of Bell's monograph was his belief that understanding how anatomy related to facial expression would allow artists to better represent emotion. This was an idea that could be traced back to the dissections of Leonardo da Vinci and Michelangelo as they tried to improve their art. He analysed in detail the way the facial muscles worked to produce different emotions, observing that it was never a single muscle at work, but groups causing changes throughout the face. If his brother had thought that the artist too often smoothed the harshness from anatomy, Charles Bell thought that the artist might remove personality from portraits in attempts to attain a classical ideal: '...he will be in danger of renouncing, in pursuit of ideal beauty, the truth of expression and of character.'[17] These ideas and their thorough anatomical underpinnings were applied to his representations of patients from Corunna and Waterloo. Through Bell's drawings and paintings, we learn not just about the wounds themselves, but can get glimpses of what these men were going through.

13 John Bell, *Engravings, explaining the anatomy of the bones, muscles, and joints* (Edinburgh: John Paterson, 1794), p.vii.

14 Michael Aminoff, *Sir Charles Bell: His Life, Art, Neurosurgical Concepts, and Controversial Legacy* (Oxford : Oxford University Press, 2017), p.29.

15 Aminoff, *Charles Bell*, p.32.

16 Robert Knox's biographer Henry Lonsdale notes that "Sir Charles was the greatest artistic anatomist of the day, but he failed twice, if not thrice, in his application for the Professorship of Anatomy to the Royal Academy in London." Henry Lonsdale, *Life of Robert Knox*, (London: Macmillan and Co., 1870), p.221.

17 Charles Bell, *Essays on the Anatomy of Expression in Painting* (London: Longman, Hurst, Rees, and Orme, 1806), p.3.

Bell's Depiction of Opisthotonos

The most famous of the Corunna oils shows opisthotonos,[18] a strange rictus where spasms of the back muscles throw the spine into a dramatic arch with head and heels curving back. Bell's notes to this painting tell us that this was composed from an amalgam of three men that he had observed suffering from the condition, all of whom had gone on to die from tetanus.[19] Their wounds had not resulted in immediate death, but all three men developed this distinctive arch, a late and inevitably fatal feature of tetanus. On the battlefield *Clostridium tetani*, a bacterium commonly found in soil and animal manure, was easily transferred into a wound. It was frequently fatal, and in 1809 there was no treatment. French military surgeon Dominique Jean Larrey advocated early amputation to minimise the chance of spread, having watched the way that opisthotonos could result several days after the development of dead tissue around a wound.[20] Many disagreed, with Bell himself writing in the second edition of *A System of Operative Surgery*, that 'the French surgeons accuse us of deferring our field operations of amputation too long, and by that losing our patients.'[21] Amputation was itself risky, and traumatic for the patient in this era before anaesthesia. Instead, tetanus patients would be sedated with opium or laudanum, and antispasmodics such as camphor rubbed into their legs and backs. In Bell's painting we can clearly see the agony of the condition.

Bell's Depictions of Resignation and of Death

Bell's painting 'Gunshot wound to the shoulder' shows pained resignation. We see a man with a gunshot wound to the right shoulder, staring blankly down, his mouth loose.[22] This is a soldier exhausted and worn down by what he has experienced. The ball had shattered the head of the humerus, passing through to injure an underlying rib. Amputation would have been the usual treatment, although Bell felt that in a patient like this – 'sunk from the loss of blood' – amputation was 'too bold.'[23] His painting shows a man exhausted by his pain and loss of blood staring at an inevitable end.

Bell also depicts death, to which he explicitly refers in the 1824 edition of *Essays on the Anatomy and Philosophy of Expression*:

18 Collection of the Royal College of Surgeons of Edinburgh, accession number GC.13842
19 Quoted in Crumplin and Starling, *A Surgical Artist at War*, p.27.
20 P. N. Skandalakis et al., '"To Afford the Wounded Speedy Assistance": Dominique Jean Larrey and Napoleon.' *World Journal of Surgery* 30 (London: 2006), pp.1392–1399.
21 Charles Bell, *A System of Operative Surgery Founded on the Basis of Anatomy.* (London: Longman, Hurst, Rees, Orme, and Brown, 1814) p.442.
22 Collection of the Royal College of Surgeons of Edinburgh, accession number GC.13835
23 Bell's notes to the case, quoted in Crumplin and Starling, *A Surgical Artist at War*, p.7.

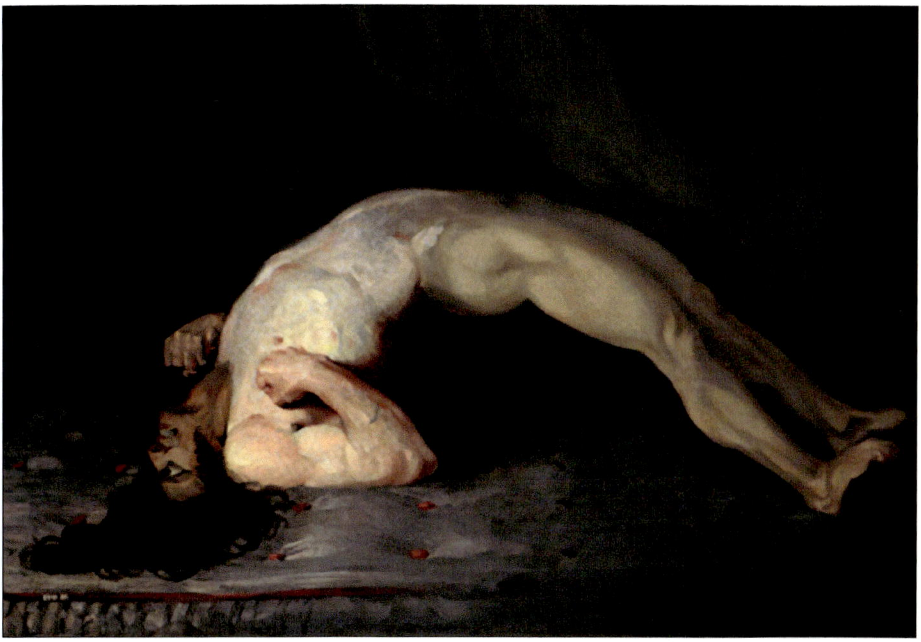

Opisthotonos, by Charles Bell. (Reproduced courtesy of Surgeons' Hall Museums, Royal College of Surgeons of Edinburgh)

> When a soldier is desperately wounded by gun-shot, or when amputation, or any other great operation of surgery is performed, a class of obscure symptoms sometimes arise, and the man dies, without the proximate cause of his death being comprehended... There is no violent pain, no cough, no inflammatory pulse; you observe only a tremulous motion and swelling of the upper lip, and working of the muscles of the nostrils. Called to him by this sign, you find his voice feeble and his words cut; and with symptoms no more marked than these, he dies.[24]

Bell has painted a man who died 12 days after receiving a wound to the chest.[25] As well as the painting itself, Surgeons' Hall Museums also holds his scapula.[26] The musket ball is embedded in it after passing through the upper lobe of the right lung. This would have been a slow, difficult death, and afterwards Bell remarked on the huge quantity of serum trapped in the chest, commenting that it would have been much relieved by drainage.[27] Here it is the *lack* of expression that Bell has depicted.

24 Charles Bell, *Essays on the Anatomy and Philosophy of Expression.* (London: John Murray, 1824) p.xvi.
25 Collection of the Royal College of Surgeons of Edinburgh, accession number GC.13829
26 Collection of the Royal College of Surgeons of Edinburgh, accession number GC.13829-1
27 Bell's notes to the case, quoted in Crumplin and Starling, *A Surgical Artist at War*, p.24.

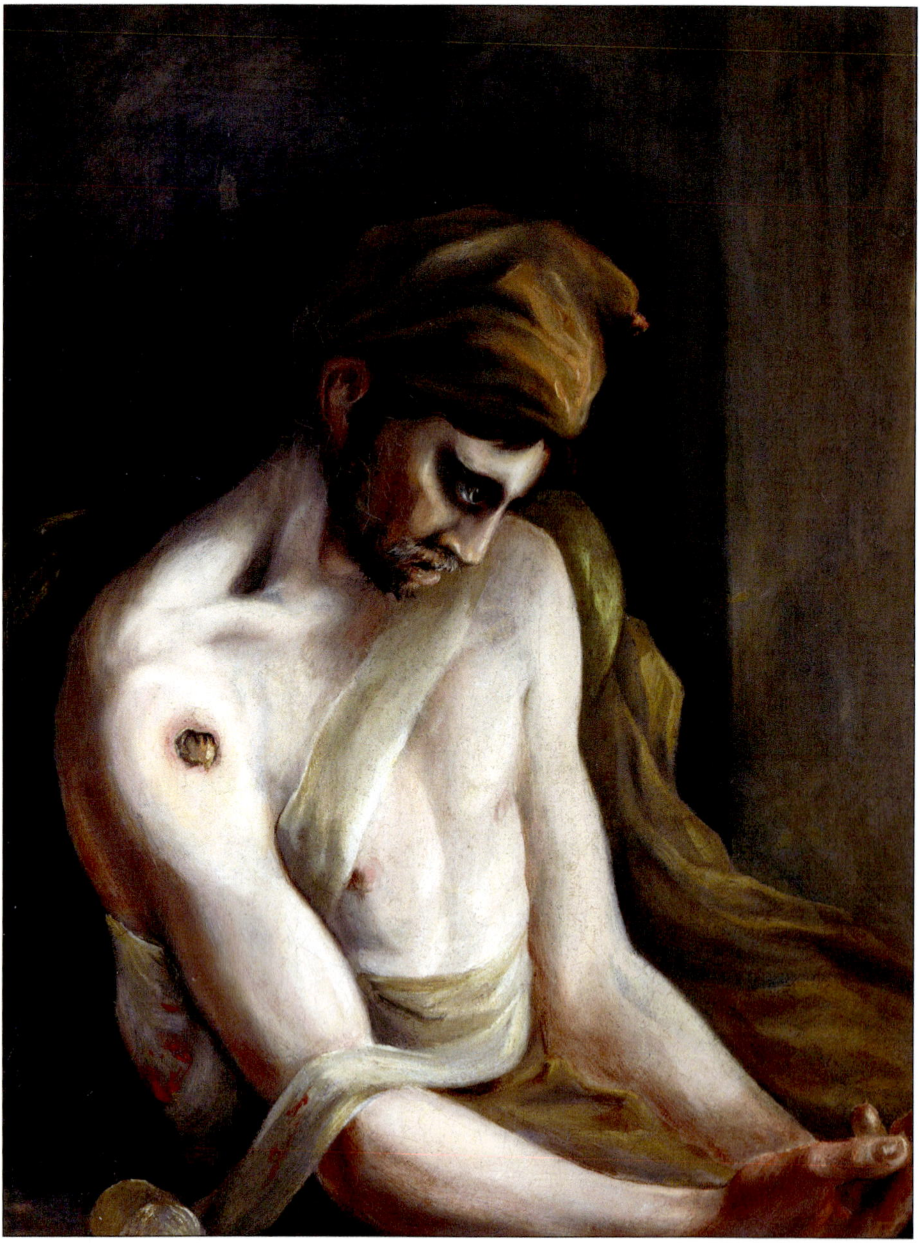

Gunshot wound to the shoulder, by Charles Bell. (Reproduced courtesy of Surgeons' Hall Museums, Royal College of Surgeons of Edinburgh)

The soldier's eyes are covered respectfully, but the lower half of his face shows the absence of muscle tension seen post mortem, the opposite of his depictions of the muscles animated by pain and emotion in life. Again, in a painting intended to teach about war injuries, we see Bell's human touch.

Bell's Waterloo Oils

Just over six years after Bell's experiences treating the wounded returning from Corunna, the Battle of Waterloo took place on 18 June 1815. Around 102,000 men were killed, injured or missing.[28] The burial of the dead in mass graves took at least 10 days. For the wounded, field hospitals were soon overwhelmed. Brussels was 12 miles away, and its six large hospitals were quickly filled. Many of the wounded were taken to Antwerp. Even for those treated in hospital, there was a shortage of surgeons. Charles Bell arrived 10 days after the battle with his brother-in-law John Shaw, 'the first professional men from England, who arrived in Brussels.'[29] Since his experience in Corunna, he had published *A Dissertation on Gun-Shot Wounds* both as an appendix to his *A System of Operative Surgery,* and in its own right.[30] The Battle of Waterloo, with its new cohort of injuries, provided Bell a prime opportunity to collect new cases – 'Johnnie, how can we let this pass?' he wrote to his brother. 'Here is such an occasion of seeing gun-shot wounds come to our very door. Let us go!'[31] His enthusiasm soon vanished as he found the suffering he saw there unbearable. 'It is impossible to convey to you the picture of human misery continually before my eyes,' he wrote to the Whig politician Francis Horner on his return to London.[32] He would end up operating for more than 12 hours per day.

> At six o'clock [in the morning] I took the knife in my hand, and continued incessantly at work till seven in the evening; and so the second and third day. All the decencies of performing surgical operations were soon neglected; while I amputated one man's thigh there lay at one time thirteen, all beseeching to be taken next; one full of entreaty, one calling upon me to remember my promise to

28 Figures from Crumplin and Starling, *A Surgical Artist at War*

29 Thomas Pettigrew, 'Charles Bell,' in *Medical Portrait Gallery. Biographical Memoirs of the Most Celebrated Physicians, Surgeons, etc., etc., who have contributed to the advancement of medical science*, vols. 3–4 (London: Fisher, Son and Co., 1838) p.5.

30 The second edition of *A System of Operative Surgery, Founded in the Basis of Anatomy* was published in 1814 including his treatise on gunshot wounds, with the dissertation published separately '*...for the accommodation of the purchasers of the former edition.*' Charles Bell, *A Dissertation on Gun-Shot Wounds.* (London: Longman, Hurst, Rees, Orme and Brown,1814) p.2. Both contain a line sketch of the opisthotonos oil mentioned earlier.

31 Quoted in *Letters of Sir Charles Bell,* p.227.

32 Letter to Francis Horner, July 1815, *Letters of Sir Charles Bellv,* p.246.

> take him, another execrating. It was a strange thing to feel my clothes stiff with blood, and my arms powerless with the exertion of using the knife.[33]

A young Robert Knox, at this point was only 24 years old, was a surgical assistant at the Gens d'Armerie hospital where Bell performed those three arduous days of surgery. Knox was not kind about Bell's surgical prowess, commenting that of 12 amputations carried out by Bell after Waterloo, 'Only one of C. Bell's lived.'[34] This is probably just an example of Knox's notoriously abrasive personality; while singling Bell out, he admits that skill and attention were generally lacking in the confined rooms of this former nunnery.[35] Observing what he regarded as 'medical dilettantism' in the treatment of the Waterloo wounded would inform Knox's stern belief in the importance of a grounding in anatomy and physiology,[36] and undoubtedly influenced his role as a teacher in the decades that followed. Later, in 1825, as Museum Conservator at Surgeons' Hall, he would arrange the purchase of Bell's collection. Buried in Knox's criticisms we glimpse the difficulty of surgery in such heightened settings, which is something Bell made explicit in his *A Dissertation on Gun-Shot Wounds* published after his experiences treating the wounded at Corunna, but before the horrors of Waterloo: 'What can a lecture in a London theatre teach of this?'[37] The scale of casualties at Waterloo was vast in comparison to what Bell had already seen, and the surgeons overwhelmed by the task at hand. If Knox was not seeing the surgeons he was assisting at their best, one has to wonder if this is surprising in these conditions?

A Sabre Wound and its Effects on the Victim

Again, Bell recorded what he had seen, showing the brutal injuries this time in water-colours. One sketch shows a trooper from the Royal Dragoons with a sabre injury to the head. Sabres were mostly used from horseback, with the momentum of the charge adding to the injury caused. Several such injuries can be seen amongst Charles Bell's collection at Surgeons' Hall, both from Waterloo and the Battle of the Pyramids, 17 years earlier. They show similar wounds across the top and back of the skull, indicative of the common trajectory of the blade from a mounted assailant. In the case of this trooper, a portion of the skull had been entirely detached by the blow, with only a small portion of scalp holding it connected. He was brought to the hospital, 'insensible …. On being urged to speak, he makes a painful effort to speak but cannot.'[38] Bell

33 Letter to Francis Horner, July 1815, *Letters of Sir Charles Bell,* p.246.
34 Gordon Gordon-Taylor, *Sir Charles Bell; His Life and Times* (Edinburgh: Livingstone, 1958), p.94.
35 Lonsdale, *Life of Robert Knox,* p.9.
36 Lonsdale, *Life of Robert Knox,* p.22.
37 Bell, *A Dissertation on Gun-Shot Wounds,* p.34.
38 Bell's sketchbook notes, quoted in T. Longmore, *Description of a series of watercolour drawings executed by the late Sir Charles Bell, illustrative of wounds received at the Battle of*

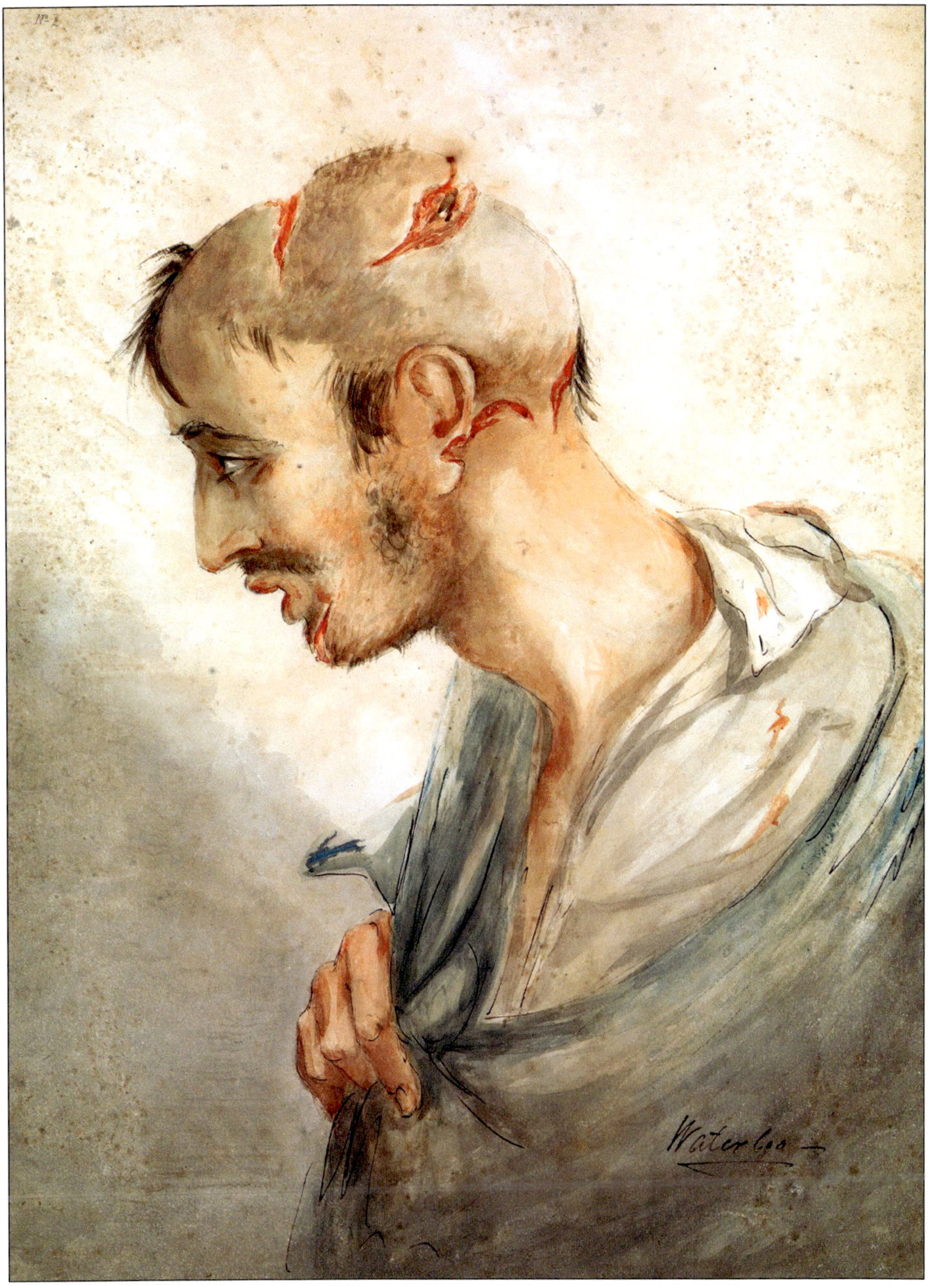

Sabre wound to head, Hôpital de la Gendarmerie, 5 July, by Charles Bell. (Reproduced with permission of Wellcome Institute Collection)

advised the removal of this fragment.[39] His watercolour depiction shows us more than just the wound. Professor of Military Surgery Sir Thomas Longmore later remarked:

> This is one of the most striking of the series of illustrations. The dull and fatuous expression of the wretched young man's countenance, and the helpless condition to which he has been reduced by the effects of the wound, are most forcibly and painfully depicted in the drawing. Not a quality which one may presume he possessed as the dragoon soldier, physical or mental remains, and the picture is distressing to gaze upon.[40]

Bell's Concern for the Wounded

Bell's correspondence after the conflict indicates the concern and care for the men he had seen. One case he had sketched showed a soldier named Voultz from the King's German Legion. His arm, according to Bell, was 'completely shattered from the elbow to the shoulder-joint.' A month and a half later, Charles Collier wrote to him from Brussels to give updates – 'In a few words, I may reply to your questions, respecting these cases.'[41] One of those is Voultz: 'I performed the operation we talked over, and I add, with gratification, successfully, i.e., it now offers every prospect of a speedy cure.'[42]

The Lasting Influence of Bell's Military Paintings

Twentieth century naval surgeon and historian Sir Gordon Gordon-Taylor considered that Bell's reputation 'rests on a very slender experience of war wounds and of surgery in the field,'[43] compared to other surgeons of the time who spent years treating the wounded from conflicts across Europe and the Americas. Bell, by contrast, spent little over two weeks of his long career in a military setting. However, Bell's experiences of Corunna and Waterloo gave rise to medical works which became standard, such as his *Dissertation on Gun-Shot Wounds*. The influence of that work can be seen in another item in Surgeons' Hall collection, this time from the American Civil War. A plaster cast shows a shoulder with a healed gunshot wound.[44] The head of the humerus had been shattered, which would often be an indication for amputation of the arm.

Waterloo. (London: Army Medical School Museum, 1866), p.7.

39 This fragment is now in the collection of Surgeons' Hall, accession number GC.12380

40 T. Longmore, *Description of a Series of Watercolour Drawings Executed by the late Sir Charles Bell* (London: Army Medical Museum, 1866), p.7.

41 Gordon-Taylor, *Sir Charles Bell; His Life and Times,* p.193.

42 Gordon-Taylor, *Sir Charles Bell; His Life and Times,* p.194.

43 Gordon-Taylor, *Sir Charles Bell; His Life and Times,* p.93.

44 Collection of the Royal College of Surgeons of Edinburgh, accession number GC.13688

The surgeon instead followed Charles Bell's teachings, and excised only the shattered bone, saving the arm. Bell's sketches in oil and watercolour were recognised for their value even more than a century later. As the First World War raged, an article in the *British Medical Journal* remarked that 'These drawings were still worthy of study as examples of the injuries sustained by our soldiers a century ago.'[45]

Charles Bell's depictions of the effects of battle are contrary to the usual depictions of war. It seems he was aware of this contradiction at the time. He talked of visiting the battlefield itself after eight days of exhausting work treating those who had been injured there. 'The view of the field, the gallant stories, the charges, the individual instances of enterprise and valour recalled me to the sense the world has of victory and Waterloo.'[46] He was constantly conscious, however, of the way his own experiences of the conflict had coloured his view of this military heroism. 'A gloomy, uncomfortable view of human nature is the inevitable consequence of looking upon the whole as I did – as I was forced to do .... there must ever be associated with the honours of Waterloo, to my eyes, the most shocking sights of woe.'[47]

Bell shows a unique perspective on the suffering of war. His sketches in oils and watercolours give us not only information about battlefield injuries, but also tell us about the human impact of the conflict on those that were there. We see men who are worn down by what they have been through and their resignation. Furthermore, Bell gives us a vision of war which is different to the heroic images presented publicly. On the 37th anniversary of the Battle of Waterloo in 1852, a triumphant equestrian statue of Wellington in bronze was inaugurated in Edinburgh, less than half a mile from Bell's Corunna oils at Surgeons' Hall. This was the usual public face of a conflict which had been victorious. Bell shows us the unsanitised horrors of war, which he is able to render more vividly through his application of anatomical knowledge to his artistic talent. This allowed Bell to contribute not only to the understanding of war injuries themselves, but also to show us the personal suffering caused by conflict.

Bibliography

Aminoff, M. J., *Sir Charles Bell: His Life, Art, Neurosurgical Concepts, and Controversial Legacy* (Oxford: Oxford University Press, 2017)

Bell, C., *Essays on the Anatomy of Expression in Painting* (London: Longman, Hurst, Rees, and Orme, 1806).

Bell, C., A *Dissertation on Gun-Shot Wounds* (London: Longman, Hurst, Rees, Orme and Brown, 1814)

45 Anonymous, 'The Middlesex Hospital School' in *British Medical Journal,* 2, 7 October, 1916 (London: 1916), p.494.

46 Letter to Frances Horner, July 1815, *Letters of Sir Charles Bell,* p.248.

47 Letter to Frances Horner, July 1815, *Letters of Sir Charles Bell,* p.248.

Bell, C. *A System of Operative Surgery Founded on the Basis of Anatomy (*London: Longman, Hurst, Rees, Orme, and Brown, 1814).

Bell, C., *Essays on the Anatomy and Philosophy of Expression,* (London: John Murray, 1824)

Bell, J., *Engravings, explaining the anatomy of the bones, muscles, and joints* (Edinburgh: John Paterson, 1794)

Cohen, J., 'Hospital Gangrene: The Scourge of Surgeons in the Past' in *Infection Control & Hospital Epidemiology,* 20;9 (London: 1999), pp.638–640

Crumplin, M. K. H. and Starling, P. H., *A Surgical Artist at War: The Paintings of Sir Charles Bell 1809–1815* (Edinburgh: Royal College of Surgeons of Edinburgh, 2005)

Gordon-Taylor, G., *Sir Charles Bell; His Life and Times* (Edinburgh: Livingstone, 1958)

Indenture between John Bell, Surgeon Apothecary in Edinburgh and Charles Bell, his brother with...Robert Bell, writer to the Signet as cautioner, Archive and Library, Royal College of Surgeons of Edinburgh (1792),

https://archiveandlibrary.rcsed.ac.uk/special-collections/incorporation-of-surgeons-and-barbers-of-edinburgh/apprenticeship-indentures-1653-1836/1230978-indenture-between-john-bell-surgeon-apothecary-in-edinburgh-and-charles-bell-his-brother-withrobert-bell-writer-to-the-signet-as-cautioner-1? (accessed 13 March 2024)

Anonymous (ed.), *Letters of Sir Charles Bell selected from his correspondence with his brother George Joseph Bell,* (London: John Murray, 1870)

Longmore, T, *Description of a series of watercolour drawings executed by the late Sir Charles Bell, illustrative of wounds received at the Battle of Waterloo* (London: Army Medical School Museum, 1866)

Lonsdale, H., *Life of Robert Knox,* (London: MacMillan and Co., 1870)

Niderost, E., 'Dismal British Retreat to Corunna' from *Warfare History Network:* (April 2009) <https://www.bing.com/search?pglt=43&q=nidersot+Dismal+British+Retreat+to+Corunna&cvid=95cf097fd2ec433e995613315042f171&gs_lcrp=EgZjaHJvbWUyBggAEEUYOdIBCDMxODhqMGoxqAIIsAIB&FORM=ANNTA1&PC=ASTS > (accessed April 18, 2024).

Oman, C., *A History of the Peninsula War* (Oxford: Clarendon Press, 1902)

Pettigrew, T. J., 'Charles Bell' in *Medical Portrait Gallery. Biographical memoirs of the most celebrated physicians, surgeons, etc., etc., who have contributed to the advancement of medical science,* vols. 3–4 (London: Fisher, Son and Co., 1838)

Skandalakis, P. N., Lainas, P., Zoras, O. et al. '"To Afford the Wounded Speedy Assistance", Dominique Jean Larrey and Napoleon' in *World Journal of Surgery,* 30 (London: 2006), pp.1392–1399

Struthers, J., 'Sir Charles Bell' in *Historical Sketch of the Edinburgh Anatomical School* (Edinburgh: Maclachlan and Stewart, 1867), pp.44–55

Anonymous, 'The Middlesex Hospital Medical School' in *British Medical Journal,* 2, 7 October 1916 (London: 1916), p.494

8

The Regius Chair of Military Surgery – the unsettling experience of military medical training at the University of Edinburgh.

Hilary S. Morris

By the early nineteenth century Scottish universities were renowned centres of learning attracting students from across Britain and beyond. New subjects such as chemistry, geology, botany, economics, and geography, which were in so many ways a direct outcome of the Scottish Enlightenment, were not only gaining in popularity but were considered to be particularly relevant by those embracing a new age defined by science and commerce. Consequently from 1790 to 1800 no fewer than 12,853 students enrolled in the University of Edinburgh alone, of whom 5,592 were in the medical faculty.[1] This too had availed itself of every opportunity to model itself on European centres of learning, particularly Leiden.[2] Along with access to the Royal Infirmary, which provided students with the patients who were required for a new type of training predominantly based on clinical diagnosis, they also had the support of a modern curriculum which included natural history, *materia medica*, anatomy, chemistry and botany. This approach to the teaching of medicine and surgery became standard practice across all Scottish medical schools and many students once qualified became particularly adept practitioners. Indeed, the Scottish medical model, as it became known, was increasingly associated with a standard of excellence and modernity, with an ability to adapt and succeed in any setting, be it military or civilian.[3]

1 The Fifth Report of the Commissioners of Military Enquiry (London: 1808), p.259.
2 This was due to the fact that many Scottish medical staff had trained in such places and therefore understood the importance of replicating this in Scotland.
3 David Hamilton, *The Healers: A History of Medicine in Scotland* (Edinburgh: Canongate,1981), p.129

Medical and Surgical Care of Military Sick and Wounded

However, the role of Scotland and its approach to medical education was to take on a particularly important role in the early years of the nineteenth century when the University of Edinburgh was selected to hold the first Regius Chair in Military Surgery, with the aim of raising the standard of medical and surgical care of sick and wounded British troops. This was a greatly needed and long overdue innovation despite the earlier work of army physician Sir John Pringle (1726–1809), who implemented preventative health measures in an attempt to improve the appalling conditions of camps and barracks. However, his achievements remained only partially effective, as the majority of medical military staff, unlike their European counterparts, took up their posts with only the briefest understanding of the specific nature of the demands they faced as medical officers. For this reason, more British troops continued to die from disease than from action on the battlefield.

Consequently, by the early nineteenth century there was an increasingly urgent call to redress this situation. Not only was the poor state of health of troops increasingly seen to be a threat to national security but it also had the potential to undermine the country's plans for colonial expansion. A government enquiry was held in 1807 tasked with reviewing the existing medical provision and finding ways of translating this into successfully maintaining the health of troops. The report of the commissioners' findings was published the following year.[4] This was a very public condemnation of the failings, particularly of the Army Medical Board, accompanied by an extensive list of explanations as to why the state of health of the troops was so poor. To improve the situation, the commissioners called for specific training for medical officers prior to their first posting. They further suggested that this could take place in general hospitals or in military establishments such as the York Hospital where newly trained medical staff would be instructed in the ways of army life and thereby be in a position to deliver a more effective model of medical care and preventative health.[5]

The sense of urgency relating to these changes was unquestionably heightened by the ill-fated Walcheren expedition of 1809 when over 4,000 British soldiers died from disease compared to the 106 who were killed in battle [6] A disaster on this scale initiated a House of Commons Enquiry which took place in 1810. Although the blame was eventually attributed to medical aid arriving too late, as opposed to gross inefficiency, there were few who failed to see that this was a situation which had every chance of being repeated unless the health of British troops was given urgent priority. It was such a concern that led to a number of medical officers taking the opportunity to present what they saw as the most effective way to implement change.

4 The Fifth Report of the Commissioners of Military Enquiry (London: 1808).
5 The Fifth Report of the Commissioners of Military Enquiry (London: 1808). p.85
6 Catherine Kelly, *War and the Militarization of British Army Medicine, 1793–1830*, vol. 5, Studies for the Society of the Social History of Medicine (Oxford: Routeledge, 2016). p.32

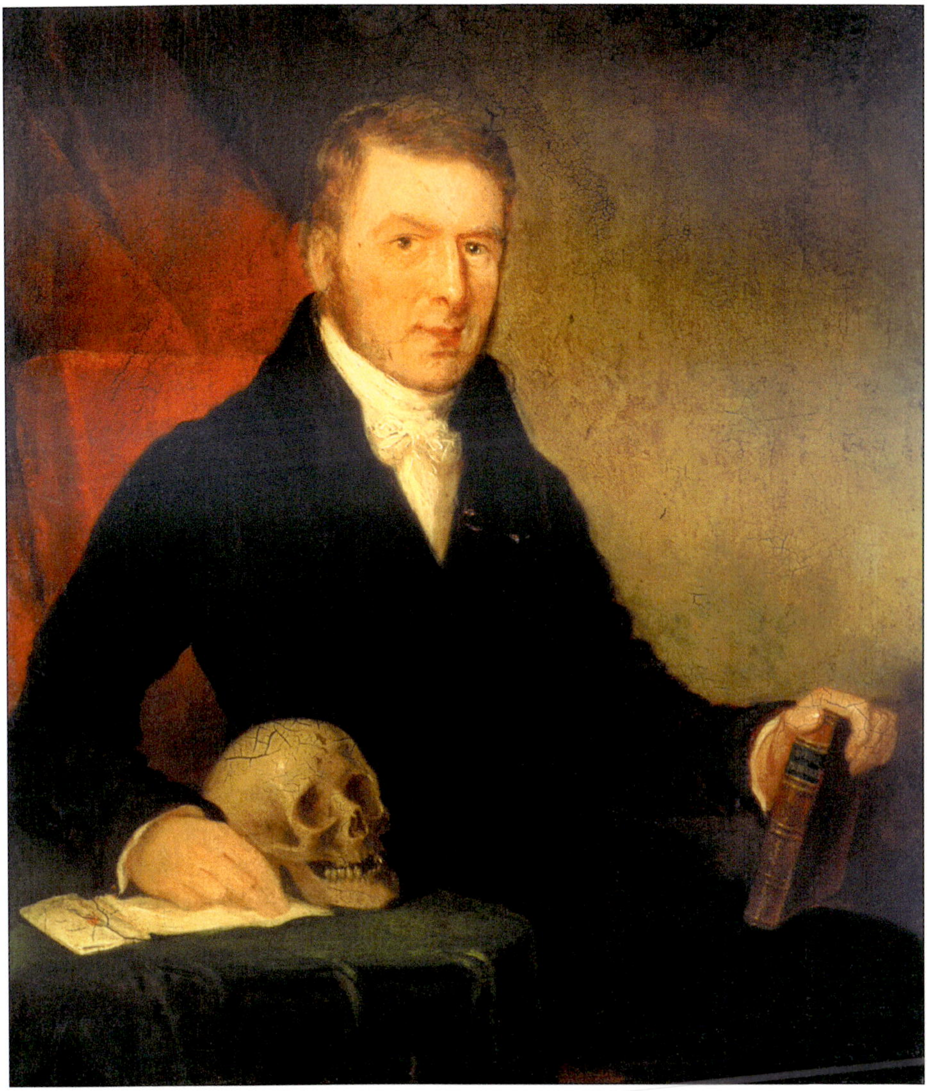

John Bell (1763–1820), Scottish surgeon. Unknown artist, *c.* 1801. (National Portrait Gallery, London, Creative Commons Attribution 3.0)

Creation of the Regius Chair of Military Surgery

One of the first to respond was the Edinburgh surgeon John Bell, who as early as 1798 had presented the idea of a school of military surgery to Earl Spencer, First Lord of the Admiralty.[7] When he failed to receive any acknowledgement, Bell took the decision to publicly address the issues by publishing his concerns regarding the state of military and naval care, along with plans for improvement. His idea was to create a school, under the auspices of a university, which would train specialist military and naval medical staff, and thereby protect Britain's security. Bell further suggested that all training should take place in a specialist building, with dissection rooms, library, access to clinical training in a nearby hospital, but still be placed in a civilian university, arguing that this type of training would ultimately benefit all of society. Not surprisingly however, with considerable finances now being invested to ensure a British victory in the war with France, innovations such as this were seen as unnecessary and costly, so were not implemented. The same response also applied to the ideas of another Scot, Robert Jackson, the Inspector General of Hospitals who was an outspoken critic of the state of military medicine and suggested the creation of a military medical training school, which was to be based either in London or on the Isle of Wight.[8]

As the war against France showed little sign of drawing to a close, the state of health of British troops, and the need to implement the most successful models of the type of surgery which aimed to see troops effectively return to the battlefield, was once again a priority. This time the eminent Scottish surgeon and physician Dr John Thomson (1765–1846) found his ideas being more favourably received. In this instance Thomson's own reputation was greatly helped by having as his patron, General Sir Thomas Maitland, who had personal experience of the dangers of sickness amongst his army. In 1797 he had to agree a truce with the Haitian leader Toussaint Louverture when plans to take the French colony of Saint Dominque failed due to vast numbers of British soldiers falling victim to yellow fever. Thomson had also previously delivered a highly successful course of lectures for additional training on all aspects of military surgery and medicine in Edinburgh between 1803–1805. There is no known evidence of Maitland being directly involved when Thomson took the decision to send these lectures as a prospectus to the army Surgeon General, Thomas Keate, though it is likely that he hoped that his plans would meet with a favourable response at the highest levels of the Army Medical Board. Moreover, continued silence from Keate now led Maitland and Spencer in 1806 to encourage Thomson to apply for a

7 John Bell, *Memoir on the Present State of Naval and Military Surgery. Addressed to the Right Honourable Earl Spenser, First Lord of the Admiralty* (Yarmouth: 1798.)

8 Robert Jackson, *An Outline of the History and Cure of Fever, Epidemics and Contagion, More Especially of Jails, Ships and Hospitals and the Yellow Fever. With Observations on Military Discipline and Economy, and a Scheme of Medical Arrangement for Armies* (Edinburgh: Printed for Mundell & Son, 1798).

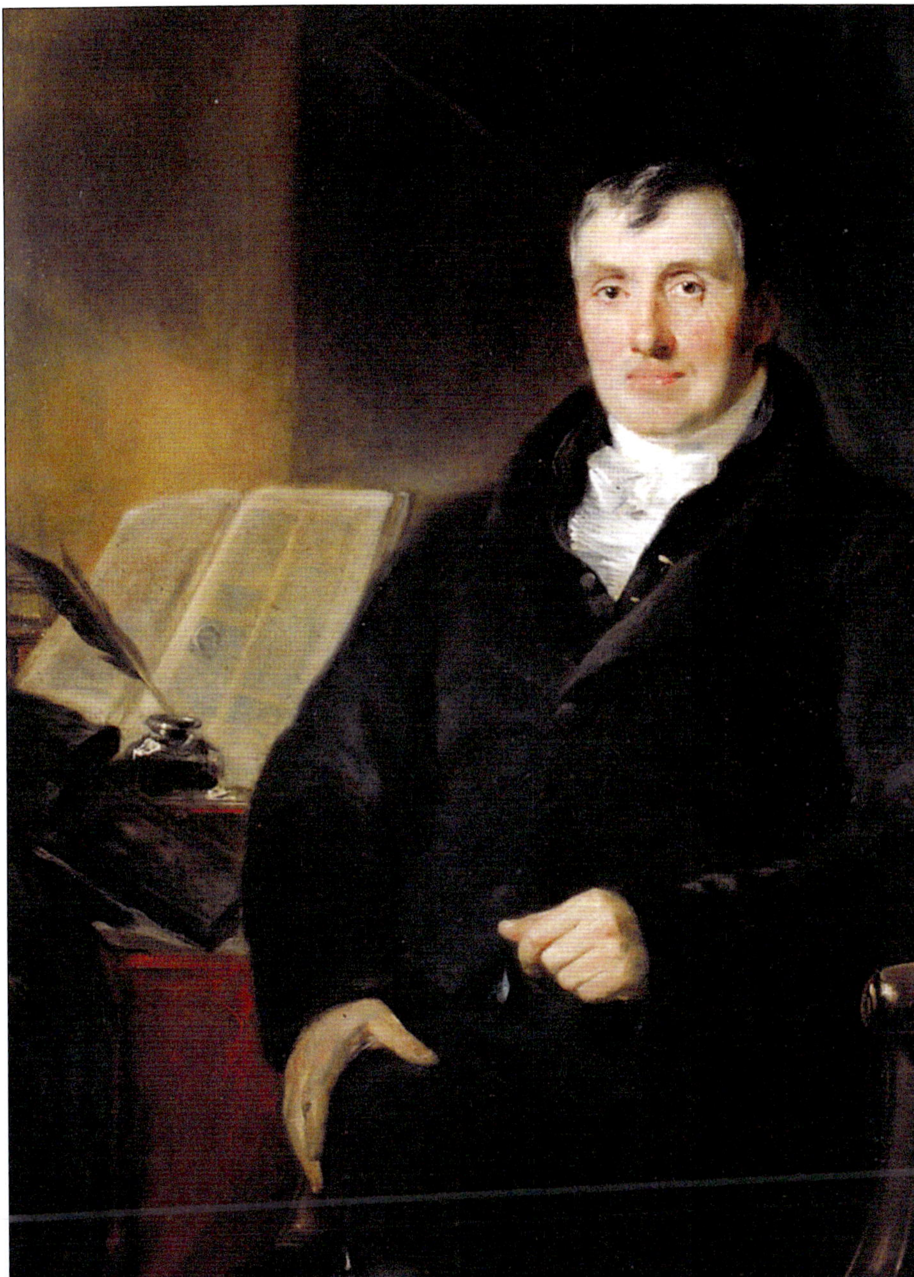

John Thomson (1765–1846), Regius Professor of Military Medicine. Portrait by Andrew Geddes, 1820. (Collection of the Royal College of Surgeons of Edinburgh. Public domain)

commission in the army, thereby placing him in the best position to implement long awaited changes should they arise. In reality this was nothing less than a plan for the creation of a new role, namely Professor of Military Surgery. Furthermore, with the continued threats of sickness along with its potential to undermine the status of the British military, in the same year George III was persuaded to grant the first Regius Chair in Military Surgery, with Thomson being appointed its first and most suitable professor. As to its location, it was announced that this would be accommodated within the University of Edinburgh.

Opposition from the University of Edinburgh

Unfortunately, the response from Edinburgh University was far from favourable. Being a Crown appointment, the university Senate had no involvement in the process, and the medical faculty were equally affronted and argued that it would have been more beneficial to all to create a new Chair of Surgery where both military and civilian needs could be addressed as a shared specialism. Consequently, Thomson began his new role not only in a hostile academic environment but also one where faculty staff went so far as to ensure that he was denied access to the teaching rooms. [9] The army too were uncomfortable with the creation of this new post and likewise denied his request for access to the military hospital in Edinburgh Castle where he planned to introduce students to the specialist training of wounds inflicted in battle.

Nevertheless, Thomson continued to promote his subject despite these setbacks. While the majority of Thomson's students were from a military background, his course was open to civilian students, in his belief that they may at some point pursue a military or naval commission. His courses therefore attracted a growing number of students and were increasingly popular. However, despite this success Thomson's position was never secure within the university. The Senate continued to make representation to have the Regius Chair removed from the University of Edinburgh and Thomson continued to be denied membership to the medical faculty as evidence that staff were not prepared to see him as one of their own, despite his medical reputation and his many professional appointments across the city. It is therefore impressive that in such a hostile environment Thomson remained in post until 1822. This was undoubtedly due to his genuine commitment to military medicine; for example in 1811 he wrote to the Army Board informing them of his decision to include additional lectures on diseases specific to different countries.[10] In 1815 he was also made Surgeon to the Forces providing him with a wealth of experience which informed his own teaching and reinforced his reputation amongst his students. It is estimated from various lecture

9 Matthew H. Kaufman, *The Regius Chair of Military Surgery in the University of Edinburgh, 1806–55* (Amsterdam: Rodopi, 2003).

10 Anonymous, *Biographical Notice of John Thomson*, p.34.

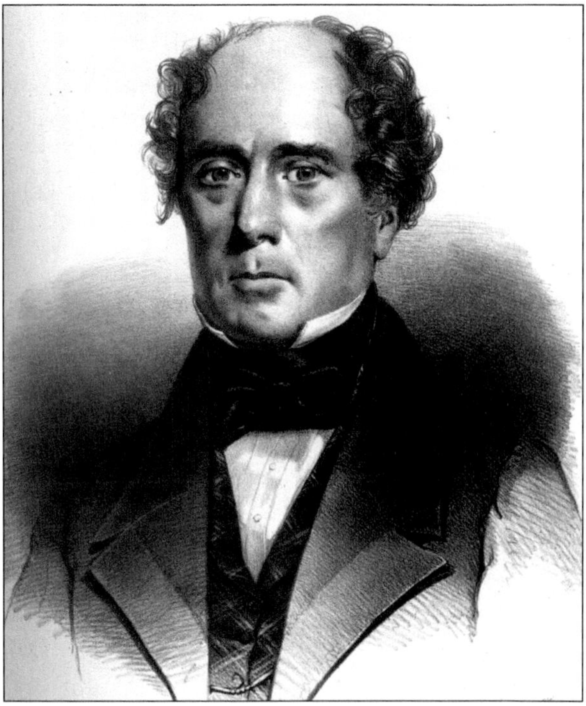

George Ballingall (1780–1855), Regius Professor of Military Surgery. Unknown artist and date. (Wellcome Collection, London. Creative Commons Attribution 4.0 International)

records that after 1815 over 250 students regularly attended his lectures.[11] In 1816 Thomson was finally given access to the military hospital though this was quickly followed by orders restricting attendance only to those students who already held a commission.

However, despite these successes Thomson faced sustained opposition from the university and his own position became increasingly untenable. In particular, he was keenly aware of the continual refusal to allow him membership of the medical faculty which he considered to be his by professional right. He therefore resigned from the Regius Chair in 1822 in the hope that he would now be regarded as the best candidate for the Chair of Physic, although this too was denied and bought to an end Thomson's association with the university. However his successor was appointed only eight days after his resignation, which suggests that the university had undergone a change in the way they viewed the Regius Chair.[12] This was certainly the result of the university now being allowed to select the next appointment on their own terms and consequently the Scottish surgeon and physician George Ballingall (1780–1855) was speedily awarded the role as the second Professor of Military Surgery. The announcement was made without opposition from any party and Ballingall commenced his new role, remaining in post until his death in 1855. During this time Ballingall was as deeply committed to the role as his predecessor and under his guidance the courses continued to produce highly specialised students training for the role of military medical officers in the British Army and the Royal Navy.

11 Matthew Kaufman, *The Regius Chair of Military Surgery*, p.69.
12 Matthew Kaufman, *The Regius Chair of Military Surgery*, p.113.

The Report of the Royal Commission

It was therefore unfortunate that just as Edinburgh came to accept this prestigious Regius Chair, the university entered one of its most uncertain periods. The Senate had long been frustrated by its lack of autonomy from the controlling influence of the all-powerful Town Council, with the result that in 1824 the university initiated legal proceedings against the continuing right of this ancient body to continue to influence academic affairs. Aware that this would not be given an impartial hearing in a Scottish court, the University also directly petitioned the Home Secretary, Sir Robert Peel, requesting a Royal Commission to enquire into the validity of their concerns. Peel responded to this request and on 25 August 1826 a Royal Commission was created to report into the state of university education in Edinburgh, though Peel quickly extended the powers of the commissioners to review each of the Scottish universities. In the final report, which was published on 28 October 1830,[13] the commissioners vindicated the grievances of the University and proposed the creation of a university court to oversee all academic affairs. However, they also proposed far reaching reform throughout each Scottish university in response to what they saw as serious failings across all faculties, something which staff were not expecting.

The Report of 1830 has long been interpreted in terms of Edinburgh University establishing itself as an academic entity free from the politics of the all-powerful Town Council.[14] However, it also was one of the most comprehensive official documents to assess the university's relationship with becoming a centre of excellence in relation to military surgery. This was due to the commissioners being able to interview both Regius Professors of Military Surgery – Thomson had retired but was still willing to give evidence and Ballingall was in post. Each provided a detailed account as to how the course in military surgery had progressed during their tenures and the problems they faced. The presence of the Regius Chair was also discussed with other medical staff to evaluate whether there were any real advantages in maintaining a separate Chair in Military Surgery. Adding weight to this discussion were the views of the highly respected Scottish physician, social reformer and Professor of Medicine at the University of Edinburgh, William Pulteney Alison. When questioned, he supported the continuation of having a military surgery specialism within the University as he felt this would not be adequately covered if it were to be absorbed into the existing courses being offered in general surgery. Alison also considered the skills and knowledge of military surgery to be such that it would benefit all medical students to participate in the course.[15]

13 *Evidence, Oral and Documented Taken and Received by the Commissioners Appointed by His Majesty George Iv, July 23rd 1826; and Re-Appointed by His Majesty William Iv, October 12th 1830. For Visiting the Universities of Scotland.*

14 Matthew Kaufman, *The Regius Chair of Military Surgery*, p.9 The Town Council in Edinburgh gained considerable power and influence throughout the eighteenth and early nineteenth centuries. In addition to overseeing the administrative needs of the city it also considered the university to be subject to its needs. This only came to an end in 1830.

15 *Evidence, Oral and Documented*, p.207.

Far less accommodating were members of the Senate who remained firmly under the control of established professors such as Alexander Monro *tertius*, the Professor of Anatomy, who also taught surgery.[16] Despite the fact that he had never practised surgery, he continued to oppose the existence of a specialism in military surgery within the university, arguing that the skills and knowledge could already be found within his general surgery classes.[17] Such was his hostility towards a military specialism that he also went so far as to refuse requests to extend his own surgical course of four and a half months to a period of six months, which was necessary in order to meet both the army and navy's criteria regarding length of study.[18] This level of hostility amongst some of the most established names in the university led the commissioners to question why the university was not prepared to impose changes regarding length of study in order to comply with the needs of military students. In response, the Senate explained that should these changes be implemented, then Edinburgh University could be seen as creating a monopoly in the training of military medical officers and also impinging on the livelihood of the private extramural schools of anatomy and surgery which provided the necessary additional teaching.[19]

The commissioners were clearly having to deal with a far more complex picture in terms of assessing the validity of not just the university but also the questionable continuation of what was a highly prestigious Regius Chair. They therefore discussed the validity of specialist training received by students at Edinburgh in terms of its long-term relevance to contemporary military and naval challenges by including the views of senior staff such as Sir James McGrigor and Sir William Burnett. While both commended the level of training offered at Edinburgh, clearly the military were still uncertain as to the value of a specialist Chair in Military Surgery in a civilian university. Hence while Burnett acknowledged it was suitable for those young medical officers at the start of their military career, he also stated that when it came to those aiming for promotion to the senior ranks, the specialist training offered in Edinburgh was insufficient to meet the range, depth and time of training the Commissioning Boards now demanded.[20] Such a view allowed the army and the navy to continue to present a case for taking back the training of their own officers, in their own environment on the grounds that only along such lines would military medical officers be assured of receiving relevant training in the most appropriate setting.

16 The Monro dynasty continued to control the teaching of surgery across all of Edinburgh's educational institutions.

17 Evidence, Oral and Documented, p.274.

18 Both the army and navy required surgeons to have completed two courses in surgery, one of which had to be six months in duration.

19 *Evidence, Oral and Documented*, p.249.

20 The Promotions Board not only required the Diploma from a Royal College of Surgeons (be it London, Dublin or Edinburgh), but also two years' hospital experience, and courses in anatomy of eighteen months, practical anatomy of twelve months, chemistry of six months, *materia medica* of three months, botany of three months, surgery of six months, theory of medicine and physic of six months and practice of medicine of six months.

The University of Edinburgh was also not averse to drawing to a close their military connections as it soon appeared there were more pressing matters requiring attention. In response to the commissioners' final report, the Senate chose to ensure the survival of the university by reverting to a more traditional model of education, which would allow greater conformity with English universities. Only then, it was argued, would Scottish degrees be able to offer graduates the chance to compete for careers in all professions within Britain. Even the Faculty of Medicine did not escape the call for reform. After the defeat of Napoleon and the reopening of Europe in 1815, the number of students fell considerably, and its privileged reputation was increasingly scrutinised and questioned.

Despite such a collection of questionable evidence the commissioners nevertheless declared that not only could they find no reason for the military association not to be maintained in Edinburgh University but also considered that it should be developed to ensure it met the needs of the military.[21] In terms of the views of the University, the Regius Chair was left very much to its own devices until the death of Ballingall in 1855. Initially Peel made it known that it was his intention to appoint a third professor and in 1857 the *Edinburgh Medical Journal* announced that Surgeon-Major Matthew has accepted the position. For reasons which remain unknown, this never occurred, and this encouraged Dr Thomas Alexander Wise to present himself as the most suitable replacement. Despite possessing genuine credentials, his enthusiasm for the post led to him privately publishing a book containing 22 testimonials endorsing his surgical skills, but his application was unsuccessful and both the military authorities and the Senate took the continued vacancy as an opportunity to effectively remove the Chair of Military Surgery by default.[22]

In order to ensure that the Chair would permanently be removed from Edinburgh, James Syme, Professor of Clinical Surgery, wrote in person to Lord Panmure, the Secretary of State for War, demanding the removal of any future government funding, fully aware that the Senate would rigorously oppose any suggestion that they take over the administrative cost of the Chair. Despite the campaign to have the Chair of Military Surgery permanently removed from Edinburgh now gaining momentum across the university, an unexpected source of contention relating to its feasibility arose through the reported actions of Ballingall and his role in the failings of the Army Medical Department during the Crimean War. He had played a prominent administrative role in the Army Medical Department for much of the war and, following the publication of a new military handbook on the construction of hospitals, was considered to be an expert in preventative health.[23] Nevertheless he was posthumously held to be responsible for many of the failings of the medical staff, an allegation which

21 Evidence, Oral and Documented, p.61

22 T. A. Wise, *Testimonies in Favour of T.A. Wise: Candidate for the Chair of Military Studies in the University of Edinburgh* (Edinburgh: Murray & Gibb, 1855).

23 George Ballingall, George, *Observations on the Site and Construction of Hospitals* (Edinburgh: Maclachan & Stewart, 1851)

famously attracted public indignation. His position as Professor of Military Surgery was likewise scrutinised for its flaws, albeit in a most unsubstantiated and unfair way.

Internal Specialisation

The army and the navy responded to the removal of the Regius Chair in Edinburgh by finally taking the opportunity to enhance their own centres of training. The Admiralty subsequently developed Haslar Hospital both as a hospital and as a training institution with its own library and museum, and in doing so, made the Edinburgh option appear both inconsequential and redundant. The situation in the army was more ambiguous. Despite the increasing number of military hospitals and an extensive series of reforms instigated by men such as McGrigor, little could be centralised in terms of training until the completion of Netley Hospital in 1863. [24] However, prior to its opening, the army, unlike the navy, did attempt in 1851 to once again establish a Chair in Military Surgery, though this time in Dublin. On this occasion it was awarded to Dr Thomas Joliffe Tufnell (1819–1885) who had established his reputation as an army surgeon at Chatham. In Dublin he taught a series of lectures on military surgery based on his experience as a medical officer in India, Ireland, and Crimea, and was known for his design for a bullet extractor which became widely used. However despite the popularity of his courses, the appointment was ended in 1860, when all training became centralised in Netley.[25]

Conclusion

In assessing the role of the Regius Chair in Military Surgery, it seems that while this was a genuine attempt to provide specialist training, it had little chance of being successful because of two contributing factors. The first was the failure of the military authorities to fully commit to the idea while it had close associations with civilian universities. The second problem was scale of reform and the type of training required was simply too vast to be addressed in this piecemeal way and the sad reality was that the health of troops did not begin to significantly improve until the early twentieth century. Nevertheless, during the 49 years of its existence, the Regius Chair of Military Surgery was led by two distinguished professors and the students they inspired may be traced throughout the years which followed as influential military medical officers many of whom rose to meet the challenge of caring for the men under their charge in the most humane and effective way possible.

24 Philip Hoare, *Spike Island. The memory of a Military Hospital* (London: Fourth Estate, 2001), p.110.

25 Neil Cantlie, *A History of the Army Medical Department* (Edinburgh & London: Churchill Livingstone, 1974), vol. 2, p.435.

Bibliography

Books

Anonymous, *Evidence, Oral and Documentary, Taken and Received by the Commissioners Appointed by His Majesty George IV. July 22nd, 1826; and Re-appointed by His Majesty, William IV, October 12th 1830: For Visiting the Universities of Scotland. Vol. 1 University of Edinburgh. Presented to both Houses of Parliament by Command of His Majesty* (London: W. Clowes & Sons, 1837)

Army Medical Department, *Fifth Report of the Commissioners of Military Enquiry* (London: 1808)

Ballingall, George, *Observations on the Site and Construction of Hospitals* (Edinburgh: Maclachan & Stewart, 1851)

Bell, John, *Memoir on the Present state of Naval and Military Surgery. Addressed to the Right Honourable Earl Spencer, First Lord of the Admiralty* (Yarmouth: 1798)

Bell, John, *Memorial Concerning the Present State of Military and naval Surgery, Addressed Several years ago to the Right Honourable Earl Spencer, First Lord of the Admiralty and now Submitted to the Public* (Edinburgh: Longman & Rees,1800)

Cantlie, Neil, *A History of the Army Medical Department*, 2 vols (Edinburgh & London: Churchill Livingstone, 1974)

Hamilton, David, *The Healers; A History of Medicine in* Scotland (Edinburgh: Canongate,1981)

Hoare, Philip, *Spike Island. The memory of a Military Hospital* (London: Fourth Estate, 2001)

Jackson, Robert, *An Outline of the History and Cure of Fever, Epidemics and Contagion, More Especially of Jails, Ships and Hospitals and the Yellow Fever. With Observations on Military Discipline and Economy, and a Scheme of Medical Arrangement for Armies* (Edinburgh: Printed for Mundell & Son, 1798)

Kaufman, Matthew H, *The Regius Chair of Military Surgery in the University of Edinburgh*, 1806–55. (Amsterdam: Rodopi, 2003)

Wise, T.A, *Testimonies in Favour of T.A Wise: Candidate for the Chair of Military Studies in the University of Edinburgh* (Edinburgh: Murray & Gibb, 1855)

Journal Articles

Kelly, Catherine, 'War and the Militarization of British Army Medicine, 1793–1830' in *Studies for the Society of the Social History of Medicine*, vol. 5 p.32

9

Dr James Barry; 'A Most Hardened Creature'

Pete Starling

Introduction

The British Armed Forces today champion equality, inclusion and diversity, to ensure that those serving in the Army Medical Services can achieve high rank regardless of gender.[1] This was not the case until the mid-twentieth century before which women were barred from serving in the army in the field of medicine, and they could not enter medical schools until the late nineteenth century.

This chapter describes a graduate of Edinburgh University who would go on to achieve both fame and high rank in the Army Medical Department.

On 25 July 1865 Inspector General of Hospitals James Barry died at 14 Margaret Street London, aged 'about 70 years'. The cause of death was given as diarrhoea, which was not in itself unusual as there was an epidemic of diarrhoea in the city at that time. The slight, effeminate James Barry was well known in military circles but he was about to become better known and secure his place in military and medical history.[2]

A Bleak Future

Born in Cork, Ireland 'about 1799', Margaret Anne Bulkley was the daughter of Mary and Jeremiah Bulkley, a grocer who had accrued many debts. Sometime in her early teens Margaret and her mother went away for some time and when they returned it was with a young baby girl. It is believed that Margaret had suffered a serious assault and been raped some time previously and this was her child, who was subsequently

1 Ministry of Defence, *A Force for Inclusion. Defence Diversity and Inclusion Strategy 2018–2030/*

2 Michael du Preez & Jeremy Dronfield, *Dr James Barry, a Woman Ahead of Her Time* (London: Oneworld, 2016)/

named Juliana. This child would eventually be given up by Margaret, but she would carry the marks of having borne her daughter (*striae gravidarum*) for the rest of her life.

With the family now in great debt and the father, Jeremiah, in prison, Margaret looked to her future and considered what to do in life. Mary and Margaret took many trips to London to elicit help from potential benefactors including Mary's brother, the artist James Barry. He initially refused to help but latterly became very supportive and so Mary and Margaret remained in London to consider what Margaret could do to try to alleviate their plight.

Gradually their fortunes started to improve and they began to move in better social circles including the medical fraternity, following introductions by Mary's brother. Medicine was a profession barred to women, but between them they hatched a plan that if Margaret disguised herself as a man, she might be able to gain entry to a medical school. To study medicine was not cheap but Margaret chose to use the inheritance from the estate of her now recently deceased uncle, James Barry, while also choosing to adopt his name. Margaret would become James Barry. Why medicine? The decision to train as a doctor may have been influenced by one of Margaret's patrons, the Venezuelan revolutionary, General Francisco Miranda.[3] Margaret would be able to use his extensive library to aid her studies, and it has been said that it was his suggestion she would become a doctor and then join him in his forthcoming revolution to liberate Venezuela from Spanish rule.[4] Margaret would never achieve that aim. After Miranda was captured and transported to Cadiz, he died there on 14 July 1816 after three years in prison. As for Margaret she took the decision to present herself as male and became known as James Barry. James and his mother sailed from Wapping to Edinburgh in late November 1809, arriving at Leith five days later.[5]

James Barry entered the University of Edinburgh in November 1809, to start one of the most demanding and rigorous courses leading to a medical qualification. This would make Barry in his early teens when he first joined the University. No doubt Edinburgh was chosen because at the time it was regarded as one of the finest medical schools in the English-speaking world and it was far away from London which would help protect his new identity. Barry also had another patron in Scotland, the 11th Earl of Buchan, who had been in the artistic circle of his uncle James Barry.

Barry initially enrolled in classes for chemistry, anatomy, surgery, natural philosophy and Greek and later added anatomical dissection and further surgery lectures. He diligently attended other extra lectures as detailed in his university record. His summer vacations were spent at Lord Buchan's home, firmly ensconced in his library.

Barry and his 'Aunt', as Mary was known, lived in various lodgings in Edinburgh. He did not mix socially with the other students who tended to regard this slight,

3 https://en.wikipedia.org/wiki/Francisco_de_Miranda; Karen Racine, *Francisco de Miranda: A Transatlantic Life in the Age of Revolution* (Wilmington: DE, Scholarly Resources, 2003)
4 du Preez, Dronfield, *Dr James Barry*, p.55.
5 du Preez, Dronfield, *Dr James Barry*, p.62.

clean-shaven male as somewhat odd in his manner and dress, but he did befriend one fellow student, John Jobson, who was invited to their lodgings and protected Barry from the teasing of other students.

Barry underwent his final examinations (many in Latin) in 1812, completing these with his dissertation on femoral hernia which he submitted 24 June 1812. He dedicated the latter to both General Miranda and Lord Buchan.[6]

Army Medical Officer

Barry moved to London in October 1812 as a pupil dresser at St Thomas's Hospital where he attended further lectures in surgery. Debts still accrued, however, and Barry explored career opportunities in the various fields of medicine to gain more funds. Finally, he settled on the army as a career. Commissioned as a Hospital Assistant on 5 July 1813, he became an Assistant Surgeon on the Staff on 7 December 1815. Much of his military service was served under the Director General Sir James McGrigor, the great reformer of the Army Medical Services.

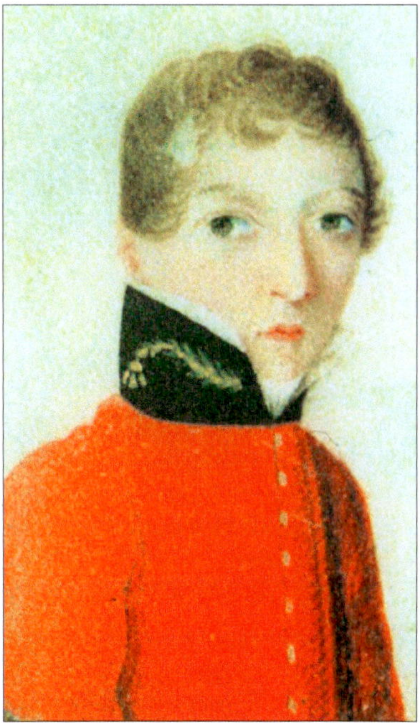

Miniature of James Barry, Assistant Staff Surgeon in uniform, *c.* 1815. (Collection of RHQ, RAMC, reproduced with permission)

Cape of Good Hope

After an initial appointment at Plymouth, he served in many parts of the world including the Cape of Good Hope and Canada, gaining a reputation as an excellent doctor but also attracting some adverse attention. Barry arrived in the Cape in late October 1816 and initially found lodgings with a widow. It was here that he enjoyed his greatest advancement in both position and medicine. Soon after arrival Barry presented himself to the Governor, the widower Lord Charles Somerset, with a letter of introduction from Lord Buchan. He quickly found favour with the Governor, initially because of his successful treatment of Somerset's very ill daughter when all else had failed. The relationship flourished and he eventually became the personal physician to Lord Charles and a great family friend. He accompanied the Governor on extended trips into the interior of the Cape, some lasting

6 James Barry, 'Disputatio Medica Inauguralis De Merocele Vel Hernia Crurali.' University of Edinburgh, thesis; 1812. https://era.ed.ac.uk/handle/1842/417

several months. Besides his work in the military hospital his private practice flourished, mainly by word of mouth, amongst the wealthy of the Cape.

On 7 December 1817 Barry was appointed Physician to the Vaccine Institute at the Cape which allowed him to receive payment to supplement his army salary, an addition not normally allowed for army surgeons. One night he was summoned to a difficult labour of a snuff merchant's wife, Wilhelmina Munnik. The midwife present could do no more and on arrival it was obvious to Barry that the only recourse was to perform the very difficult caesarean section, a procedure which almost inevitably resulted in the death of the mother and an operation that Barry had never previously performed. He performed it with great success and both mother and son survived. The son was named James Barry Munnik.

One other officer who enjoyed the Governor's favour was one of his aides-de-camp, Captain Josios Cloete, the son of an affluent local family. Barry and Cloete would meet often in the outer rooms of the Governor's office. Cloete was jealous of Barry's influence over the Governor and suspected that all was not correct with this army doctor. On one occasion while in the Governor's outer office Barry made disparaging remarks about a female visitor to the Governor's office. Cloete took exception to this and demanded Barry retract his comments, which he refused to do. Not wanting to engage in any major physical altercation Cloete stood and grabbed Barry by the nose. There was only one outcome to this insult – Barry demanded a duel. At the appointed time and place they faced each other and fired. Barry's ball struck the peak of Cleote's shako but did not cause an injury, while Cloete's ball struck Barry's thigh and caused a flesh wound. Honour was satisfied and the pair remained on good terms for many years thereafter.

His relationship with the Governor eventually caused a public scandal especially after an anonymous placard was posted publicly, accusing the Governor and Barry of being seen engaged in an unnatural sex act together. This led to a public enquiry but, despite both Somerset and Barry offering sizeable rewards, the author of the placard was never caught.

Corfu

When Barry eventually left the Cape he did so having made significant advances in public health. He arrived at Corfu in April 1851 as the Principal Medical Officer with the rank of Deputy Inspector General. Corfu at that time was home to several infantry battalions as well as artillery units, each with their regimental hospitals. He immediately set about improving the medical care of the troops with his usual vigour. In the spring of 1852 he took 10 months home leave and arrived back on Corfu on 1 April 1853.

Not long after that he attracted controversy when he was placed under close arrest after an altercation with Lieutenant Colonel William Denny, Commanding Officer of the 71st (Highland) Light Infantry. Barry was incensed that convalescents were being used on fatigues and made his feelings known, possibly striking Denny with his riding crop. Luckily for Barry the matter was not pursued and passed into oblivion as far as the army was concerned.

Crimea

As the Crimean campaign commenced and with it the large numbers of sick compared with wounds of battle, Corfu was turned into a convalescent centre with ships arriving from Scutari Hospital, Constantinople on a regular basis. Barry was not allocated a medical position in the Crimean campaign but in October 1855 he took leave of absence to travel to Constantinople to observe at first hand the treatment of the sick and wounded. He did this with his usual panache accompanied by two servants, his grey Arab horse, his dog and a goat as a source of milk.

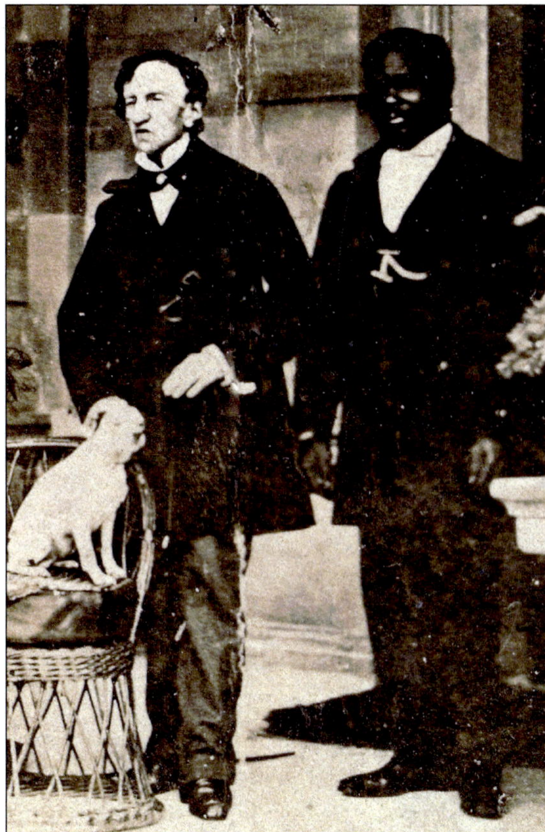
James Barry with his servant John and dog Psyche in Jamaica. (Reproduced courtesy of Museum of Military Medicine collection)

His first call was on Dr Alexander Cumming, the Principal Medical Officer at Scutari. He failed to make a good impression with Cumming who immediately wrote to John Hall, the Principal Medical Officer to warn him of Barry's impending visit. Hall always felt threatened by Barry, believing that Barry felt he should be Principal Medical Officer for the Crimean campaign, especially as Barry was two years senior to Hall.

There was one other person that Barry failed to impress at Scutari. As he entered the imposing barrack hospital quadrangle, Barry noticed a young woman, whom he thought to be a nurse, walking across the square in the blazing sun but without suitable protection on her head. Barry immediately criticised the woman at length in front of a crowd berating her for her carelessness. The object of his wrath was Florence

Nightingale, who later recalled that she 'never had such a blackguard rating in all my life'. She thought Barry 'the most hardened creature' she had ever met.[7]

Barry made his way to Balaclava and to the camp of the 4th Division. Here he stayed until January 1856 when he returned to Corfu, remaining there until 23 June 1857, when he departed for England. He then embarked for Canada in October 1857. Prior to that another conflict had broken out in India. Anxious that he would miss out on this conflict, Barry hoped that his orders for Canada would be cancelled and he would receive orders to take up a senior medical post in India. This did not happen and Barry took up his post in Canada, arriving in Montreal on 3 November 1857.

Canada

Barry set about this appointment with vigour but again attracted attention as he sped around the city in a sleigh, with footmen and dogs. His reputation was again called into question when he incurred the wrath not only of other officers but also of the clergy. He publicly berated the Bishop of Montreal because he wanted the time of the Sunday church service changed to 9am. The request was denied, hence the outburst. A letter of complaint against Barry was sent to the General Officer Commanding, Lieutenant General Sir William Eyre, resulting in Barry issuing an apology. Barry also came to the notice of Eyre over his interference in the medical board of an infantry officer. Eyre could take no more of this strange medical officer so wrote to Horse Guards requesting that Barry be recalled to England.

By this time Barry himself was ill and felt it was time to finally go home. On 14 May 1859 he boarded a ship for the long voyage to England. There he appeared before a medical board and was forced to retire from the Army in July 1859 due to age and ill health. In retirement he lived alone in London, renting rooms at a dentist's house in Marylebone.

A Sad Death

Barry died penniless and intestate on 25 July 1865. After his long-standing friend the surgeon David Reid McKinnon had certified that life was extinct, he left the room. It was then that the remarkable discovery became known. It was first thought that the body was laid out by the maidservant Sophia Bishop, although du Preez and Dronfield consider that this was done by an unnamed charlady.[8] When the body was undressed it was found to be that of a woman, one who had, in younger years, given birth. The woman laying out the body felt that she was owed money for her services.

7 Florence Nightingale to her sister, Frances Verney (undated). Welcome Library Collection MS 9001/145.

8 du Preez, Dronfield, *Dr James Barry*, pp.390–391.

Moreover, she reckoned that there was more money to be made from her discovery. After McKinnon and Barry's army agent refused to pay her anything, the story appeared in the national press both in England and Ireland and eventually attracted the attention of the General Registrar who wrote to McKinnon for clarification of Barry's sex. McKinnon replied stating that having known Barry for many years he could categorically say that Barry was a male. Yet evidence which subsequently came to light suggested otherwise.

How had Barry managed to keep this secret over all the years at medical school and military service? Was there some sort of medical examination on entry to the army? Kaufman states in *Surgeons at War* that entry requirements of the time included being free from physical defects or disease.[9] June Rose in *The Perfect Gentleman* speculates that perhaps Barry's Edinburgh degree and prior medical experience between graduation and entry to the army contributed to the exemption for the need for a physical examination,[10] and that the army was just keen to have an experienced and well-educated applicant.

There were several times throughout Barry's career when his former identity might have been revealed. As mentioned above, in 1819 Barry fought a duel with Captain Josias Cloete, aide-de-camp to Lord Charles Somerset. Cloete's ball struck Barry in the upper thigh but when the attending surgeon went to cut off Barry's trouser leg to expose the wound Barry stopped him and, back in his rooms, treated the flesh wound himself.

Also while in the Cape, when treating a female patient, Barry stayed at the patient's house. On one occasion a female nurse, also employed to look after the patient, went to Barry's room to summon him and, without knocking, opened the door to find herself faced with a female in a state of undress. From then on the relationship soured, eventually forcing the nurse to leave the Cape but keeping her secret to herself.

In 1842 Barry succumbed to fever in Port of Spain and was looked after by a female friend on the condition that should Barry die there was to be no physical examination, but the body was to be wrapped in a bed sheet and buried. His medical colleagues were ordered not to call or attend on him. One colleague however, Dr Nicholas O'Connor, ignored that request and, finding Barry asleep, pulled down the bed sheet to examine him further and found he was looking at the body of a female. Barry suddenly awoke and, finding his medical colleague in the room, swore him to secrecy for life. [11]

9 Matthew H. Kaufman, *Surgeons at War, Medical Arrangements for the Treatment of the Sick and Wounded in the British Army during the Late 18th and 19th Centuries* (London: Greenwood Press, 2001).

10 June Rose, *The Perfect Gentleman* (London: Hutchinson & Co, 1977).

11 du Preez & Dronfield, *Dr James Barry*, p.294.

A Question of Age

There has been much controversy about Margaret Bulkley's/James Barry's age.

For the death certificate McKinnon guessed the age to be 70, so given a year of death of 1865 he would have been born around 1795. Other sources state 1790 and Barry himself states 'about 1799' as the year of birth. The record of burials states 'aged 71'.

Barry went to Edinburgh in 1809 so if he was born 'about 1799' that would make his age 10 years. If he was born in 1795 then he was aged 14 years on entering medical school. He states himself that he entered the army under the age of 14 years. Brockliss et al discuss the age of medical officers on entry to the army and show that ages on appointment ranged from 14 to 49; George Guthrie was examined by the College of Surgeons on 2 February 1801 when aged 15. In March of that year he was appointed Assistant Surgeon to the 29th Regiment.

It would eventually be under McGrigor's directorship that a minimum age requirement of 21 years was introduced for medical officers.

James Barry was buried in Kensal Green Cemetery on 29 July 1865 without military ceremony as at the time such honours were conferred only on officers who died in service.

Epilogue

Barry has been commemorated in various ways by the Army Medical Services. There was a Barry Ward in the Queen Alexandra Military Hospital, Millbank during the hospital's lifetime and a Barry Room in the Headquarters Officer's Mess, next door to the hospital on Millbank. Neither of these institutions any longer exist. A watch chain purporting to have been Barry's is in the collection of the Museum of Military Medicine.

The story remains an important episode in the history of the Army Medical Services. Margaret Bulkley/James Barry was a pioneer not only in medicine but also the Army Medical Services and it was not until 1950 that female doctors were given the same status as male doctors in the army.

Bibliography

Archive Sources

The National Archives WO25/3910, Records and particulars of Professional Education – Surgeons

The National Archives WO138/1, Memorandum on the Services of Dr James Barry, Inspector General of Hospitals.

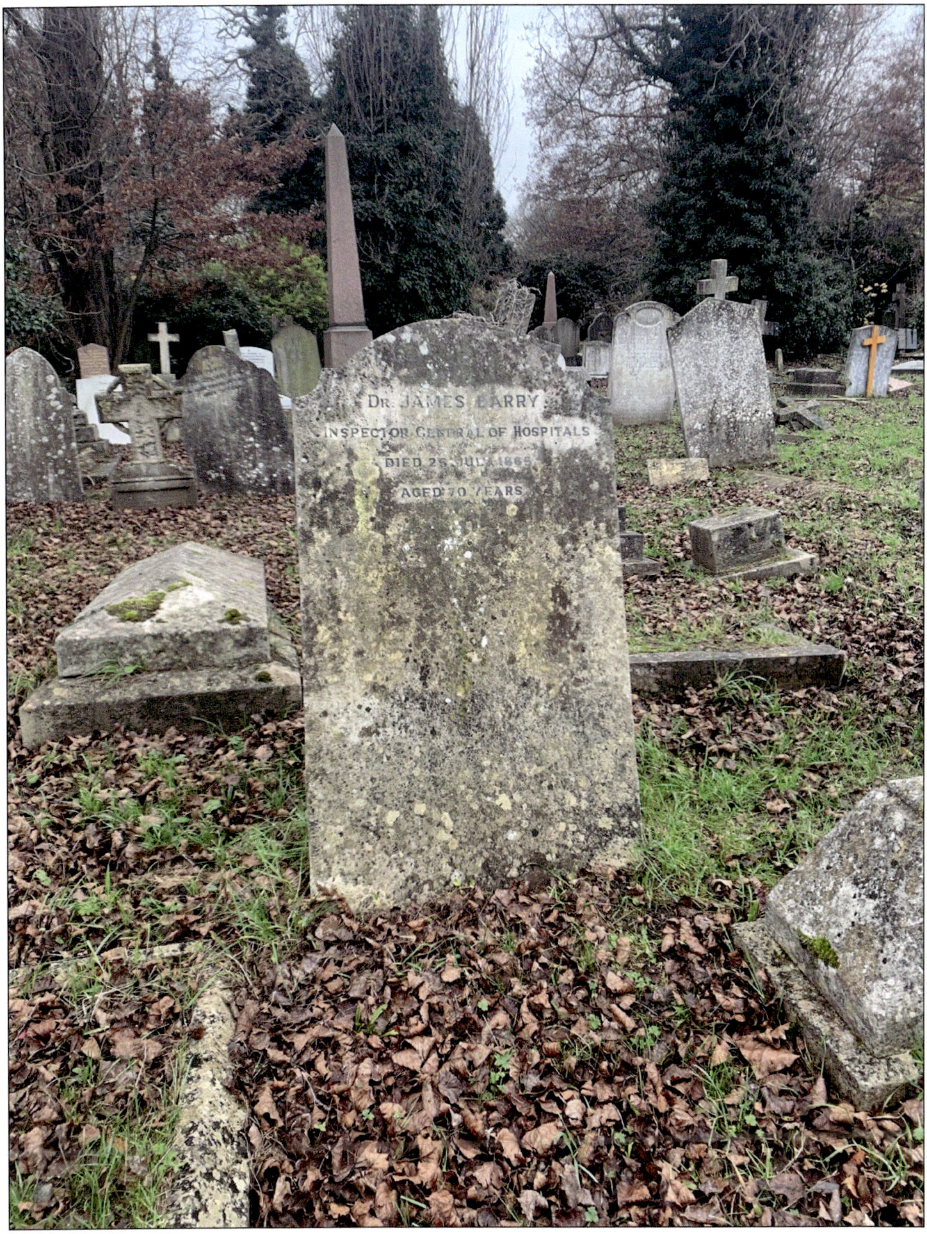

The grave of James Barry in Kensal Green Cemetery. (Author's Collection)

Wellcome Library Collection MS 9001/145, Letter (undated) Florence Nightingale to her sister Frances Verney

Primary Sources

Ministry of Defence, *A Force for Inclusion. Defence Diversity and Inclusion Strategy 2018–2030*

Secondary Sources

Brockliss, Laurence, *Advancing with the Army, Medicine, the Professions, and Social Mobility in the British Isles, 1790–1850* (Oxford; Oxford University Press 2006)

Cantlie, Neil, *A History of the Army Medical Department,* 2 vols (London: Churchill Livingstone, 1974)

Hinton, Michael, *Victory over Disease, Resolving the Medical Crisis in the Crimean War 1854–1856* (Warwick: Helion & Company, 2019)

Holmes, Rachel, *Scanty Particulars* (London: Viking, 2002)

Hurt, Raymond, *George Guthrie, Soldier and Pioneer Surgeon* (London: Royal Society of Medicine Press, 2008)

Johnston, William, *Roll of Commissioned Officers in the Medical Service of the British Army, 20 June 1727 to 23 June 1898* (Aberdeen: The University Press, 1917)

Kaufman, Matthew H., *Surgeons at War, Medical Arrangements for the Treatment of the Sick and Wounded in the British Army during the Late 18th and 19th Centuries* (London: Greenwood Press, 2001)

du Preez, Michael & Dronfield, Jeremy, *Dr James Barry, a Woman Ahead of Her Time* (London: Oneworld, 2016)

Racine, Karen, *Francisco de Miranda: A Transatlantic Life in the Age of Revolution* (Wilmington DE: Scholarly Resources, 2003)

Rose, June, *The Perfect Gentleman* (London: Hutchinson & Co, 1977)

Shepherd, John, *The Crimean Doctors*, 2 vols (Liverpool: Liverpool University Press, 1991)

Journal Article

Barnsley, R. E., 'The Diaries of John Hall, Principal Medical Officer in the Crimea, 1854 to 1856' in *Journal of the Society for Army Historical Research,* 41(London: 1963), p.165

Websites

https://en.wikipedia.org/wiki/Francisco_de_Miranda (accessed 8 January 2024)

10

Sir David Bruce and the Saga of Brucellosis

David Vassallo

Introduction

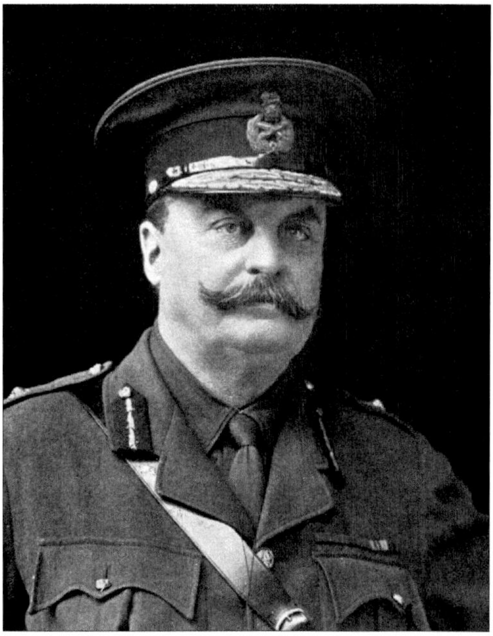

Sir David Bruce. (RAMC Muniments Collection, Wellcome Library, reproduced with permission)

I am indebted to my late father, Dr Luis Adrian Vassallo (1933–1994),[1] consultant physician from Malta, who was fascinated by the saga of brucellosis. His enthusiasm for its history, his inspiring lectures, and his shrewd insights into the personalities involved enkindled in me a similar interest. The story is so full of unexpected events, coincidences, controversy and insights into the capriciousness of human nature that it well merits description as a saga. This Chapter is based largely on my father's unpublished notes and his Sydenham lecture 'The Saga of Brucellosis', delivered posthumously on his behalf to the Worshipful Society of Apothecaries, London on 6 November 1995, and later published in part in *The Lancet*.[2]

1 D. J. Vassallo. L A Vassallo. (Obituary), *British Medical Journal* 309, (1994), p.1578.
2 D. J. Vassallo, 'The Saga of Brucellosis: Controversy over Credit for Linking Malta Fever with Goats' Milk' in *The Lancet,* 348 (1996), pp.804–808.

Brucellosis and the Island of Malta

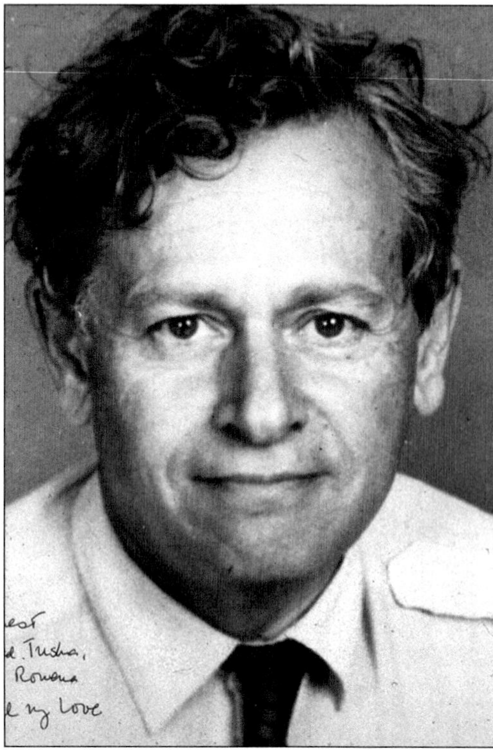
Dr Luis Adrian Vassallo, May 1994.
(Photo: author's copy)

Brucellosis, a chronic and debilitating feverish illness previously known as Malta, Mediterranean or Undulant Fever, has almost certainly plagued peoples of the Mediterranean littoral and further afield from beyond time immemorial. Its causative organism was discovered in Malta in 1887 by Surgeon Captain David Bruce (1855–1931), then a young medical officer in the British Army, though it would be another 18 years before the mode of transmission was elucidated.

British troops first arrived in Malta in 1798 during the Napoleonic Wars, helping the Maltese oust the French invaders. The British remained by invitation of the Maltese, with the Royal Navy stationing its Mediterranean Fleet in Malta's majestic Grand Harbour. Malta's strategic importance increased after the Suez Canal opened in 1869. Bruce arrived there in 1884, at the height of Empire.

The Young Bruce

David Bruce was born on 29 May 1855 in Bendigo, Australia to Scottish parents; engineer David Bruce from Airth and his wife Jane Russell Hamilton from Stirling, who had emigrated to Australia in the 1850 gold rush. When he was five years old the family returned to Stirling, where he developed a lifelong interest in natural history.[3] He entered Edinburgh University as a zoology student, transferred to medicine and graduated with distinction in 1881. Soon he became keenly interested in the scientific side of medicine, wanting to follow in the footsteps of Pasteur, Koch and Lister, but did not have sufficient funds. He therefore entered general practice in Reigate, Surrey

3 David Bruce, Lecture to medical students, Aberdeen University, 1922.

in 1881 as assistant to a Dr Stone. There he fell in love with Mary Elizabeth Sisson Steele, daughter of his partner's predecessor.[4]

Mary Elizabeth Steele was born in 1849. She was the sixth of nine children of the much-respected Reigate general practitioner, Dr John Sisson Steele, who was also a fine artist and Mary inherited his talent for accurate drawing and sketching. She would put this talent to good use assisting her future husband in the laboratory, producing thousands of drawings of microscopic organisms, many preserved in the RAMC Muniments Collection.[5]

Planning to marry, but without private means, Bruce decided to transfer to the Army:

> But as I still hankered after the scientific side of medicine I conceived the idea of going into the Army Medical Service where I would get my bread and butter, and at least there would be plenty of leisure. This I did in 1883 and early in the following year found myself stationed in Malta. There was no doubt about the leisure. The day's work could be done as a rule in about half an hour...[6]

Bruce was commissioned as Surgeon Captain in the Army Medical Department on 4 August 1883,[7] having gained first place in the entrance examination and then finishing in first place in the passing out examination at the Army Medical College, Netley that same year.[8] He could now marry Mary, which he did on 8 December 1883. On 10 March 1884 they arrived in Malta on the troopship HMS *Malabar* for his five-year tour of duty (1884–1888). Bruce was appointed medical officer in charge of the Station Hospital (previously the Sacra Infermeria of the Knights of St John) in Valletta, where he encountered the first of hundreds of Malta Fever patients.

This mysterious illness was wreaking havoc amongst the soldiers and sailors of the Malta Garrison. Bruce was familiar with the first paper on this illness published in 1863 by a British military surgeon, Assistant Surgeon Jeffrey Allen Marston. Marston gave an accurate description of the illness in troops invalided to Malta during the Crimean War, calling it "Mediterranean Remittent (or) Gastric Remittent Fever". Marston poignantly depicted his own sufferings, noting the irregular type of fever, the languor and weariness, the muscle and joint pains, the gastro-intestinal symptoms

4 Ethelwald E. Vella, 'Major-General Sir David Bruce, K.C.B.' in *Journal of the Royal Army Medical Corps,* 119 (3) (1973), pp.131–144.

5 RAMC Muniments Collection – Archives and manuscripts related to Sir David Bruce and Lady Bruce https://wellcomecollection.org/works/srscccsk (accessed 31 May 2024)

6 Bruce. Lecture to medical students.

7 Anonymous, 'Obituary, Sir David Bruce' in *Obituary notices of Fellows of the Royal Society,* 1, (1932), pp.79–85.

8 J. E. Noble, 'The David Bruce Laboratories 25th anniversary' in *Journal of the Royal Army Medical Corps* 113, (1967), pp.208–212; A. Hamerton, 'Obituary – Major-General Sir David Bruce' in *Transactions of the Royal Society of Tropical Medicine & Hygiene,* 25, (1931–1932), pp.305–312.

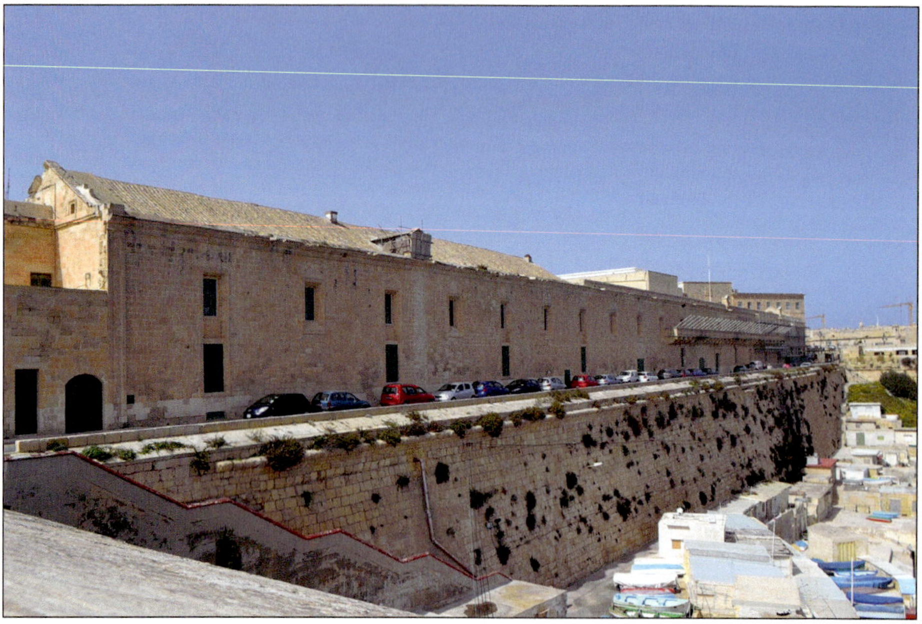

The Sacra Infermeria. (Station Hospital), Valletta (Photo: David Vassallo)

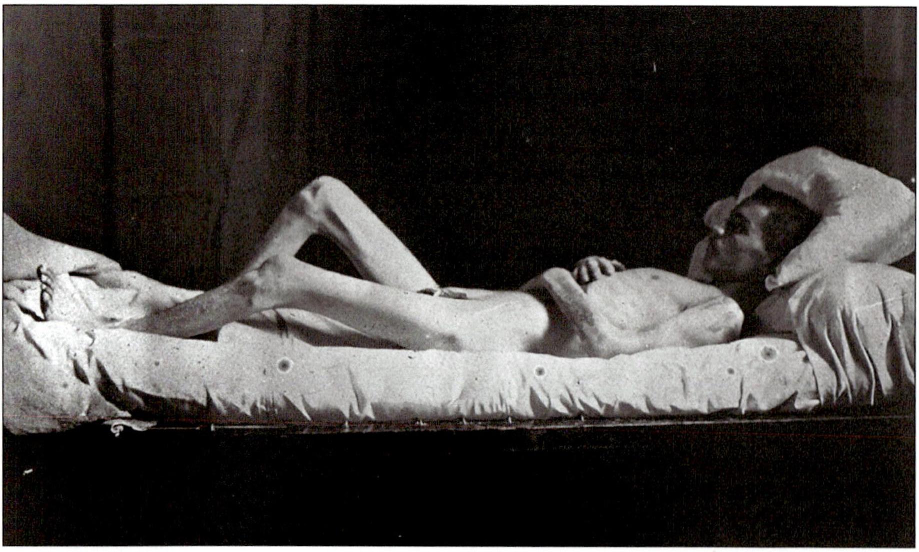

Malta Fever patient. (Photo: David Bruce, RAMC Muniments Collection, Wellcome Library, reproduced with permission)

and the long duration of illness: 'The patient is prone to relapses, and the disorder is followed by a protracted convalescence – very frequently also by rheumatism of some form or other.'[9]

The Bruces arrived in Malta at the dawn of the golden age of microbiology. Only four years previously Alphonse Laveran, a French army surgeon in Algeria, had discovered malaria parasites in the red blood cells of man, though the way in which this great scourge of mankind was transmitted was still a mystery.

The year 1884 was also when Dr Robert Koch in Berlin proved that cholera was due to a specific micro-organism, and just two years since Koch had revealed to the world the identity of the tuberculosis bacterium, the 'Captain of the Men of Death', responsible then for the deaths of one in seven human beings.

Bruce resolved to find the cause of Malta Fever. The challenges he faced were peculiar to a peacetime garrison:

> But on the other hand there was no encouragement or assistance of any kind for research work. There was no laboratory, not even a microscope in the hospital. In fact, in those days your brother officers almost looked on it as a crime if you presumed to do anything outside your strict duty. So I had to set up a laboratory and provide myself with microscope and other apparatus.... Before long I was at work trying to find out the nature of Malta Fever. [10]

Bruce was initially sceptical about Koch's findings:

> It is difficult to put prejudice aside and I can well remember in the year 1882 the scepticism with which I first heard of the new discovery, that consumption was caused by a minute vegetable parasite. It was with difficulty then that I brought myself to take up the study of Malta Fever by the new methods, but at last by the help of a neighbouring tin-smith I found myself in possession of the necessary bacteriological apparatus and started work...[11]

Bruce closely followed the methods of Koch and Gaffky, whose techniques first became readily available in English translation in the book *Microparasites in Disease* published in 1886, two years after he arrived in Malta. He acknowledged this in his 1888 article.[12]

Bruce made the first important breakthrough on Boxing Day 1886, by fulfilling the first of Koch's postulates. He identified numerous micrococci in the spleen at the post mortem examination of a young soldier, 20 year old Private John Riddall,

9 J. A. Marston, Report on Fever (Malta), *Army Medical Department Medical Report for 1861*. 3, (London: 1863), pp.520–521.
10 Bruce. Lecture to medical students.
11 Bruce. Lecture to medical students.
12 David Bruce, 'The Micrococcus of Malta Fever' in *Practitioner*, 40, (1888), pp.241–249.

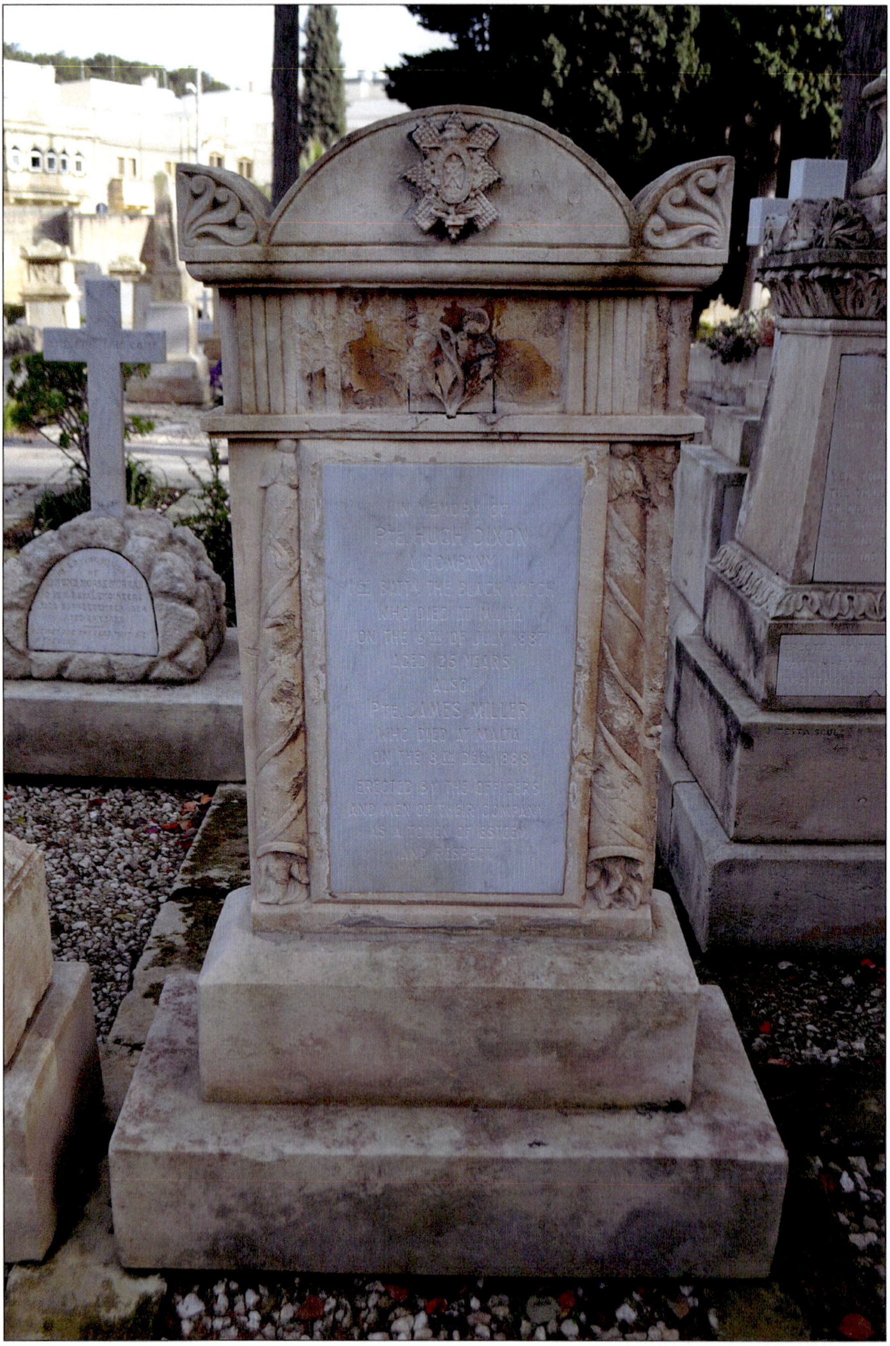

Private Hugh Dixon's grave, Pieta Military Cemetery, Malta. (Photo: David Vassallo)

2nd Battalion, King's Own Yorkshire Light Infantry, who died of Malta Fever in the Forrest Hospital, Spinola, on 26 December. Private Riddall was buried in Pieta Military Cemetery.

Bruce fulfilled the second of Koch's postulates in July 1887 when he successfully cultivated the Micrococcus in vitro, from the spleen of another young soldier who died of this illness. The unfortunate soldier whose death hereby earned him a place in medical history was 25 year old Private Hugh Dixon, 1st Battalion The Black Watch (Royal Highlanders), who died on the twelfth day of his illness, on 6 July 1887. He too was buried at Pieta.

Bruce was aided by the Maltese Government analyst, Dr Joseph Caruana Scicluna.[13] They are commemorated together on a plaque outside the Sacra Infermeria.

Bruce fulfilled the last of Koch's postulates in August 1887 by successfully infecting a monkey with the Micrococcus and cultivating the organism from its spleen. He published his findings in *The Practitioner* in 1887 and 1888. Bruce had discovered the causative organism of Malta Fever, later naming it *Micrococcus Melitensis* from the Roman name for Malta.

The Bruces left Malta at the end of 1888. In 1889 Bruce was appointed Assistant Professor of Pathology at the Army Medical School, Netley, near Southampton.

Matthew Louis Hughes

On Christmas Day, 1891, a bright young doctor who had graduated top of the class at Netley, Surgeon Captain Matthew Louis Hughes (1867–1899), arrived in Malta for a six-year tour of duty.[14] He was the great-grandson of one of Nelson's admirals, Sir Thomas Louis, and was therefore known as Louis Hughes.

The Loss of HMS *Victoria*

Two years later, on 22 June 1893, the Royal Navy suffered its greatest peacetime disaster: the collision during annual manoeuvres in calm seas off Syria between two of Her Majesty's finest battleships, the *Victoria* and the *Camperdown*, flagships of the First and Second Divisions of the Mediterranean Fleet.

This disaster resulted in the loss of the *Victoria* and most of her crew, including the Fleet's Commander-in-Chief, Britain's most renowned naval officer, Vice Admiral Sir George Tryon. The disaster resulted from Tryon's enigmatic order for the two Divisions of the Fleet to reverse course by turning inwards towards one another.

13 David Bruce, Note on the Discovery of a Micro-organism in Malta Fever. *Practitioner*, 39, (1887), pp.161–170.

14 G. W. G. Hughes and M. H. Hughes. 'Matthew Louis Hughes and Undulant Fever' in *Journal of the Royal Army Medical Corps*,115, (1969), pp.199–203.

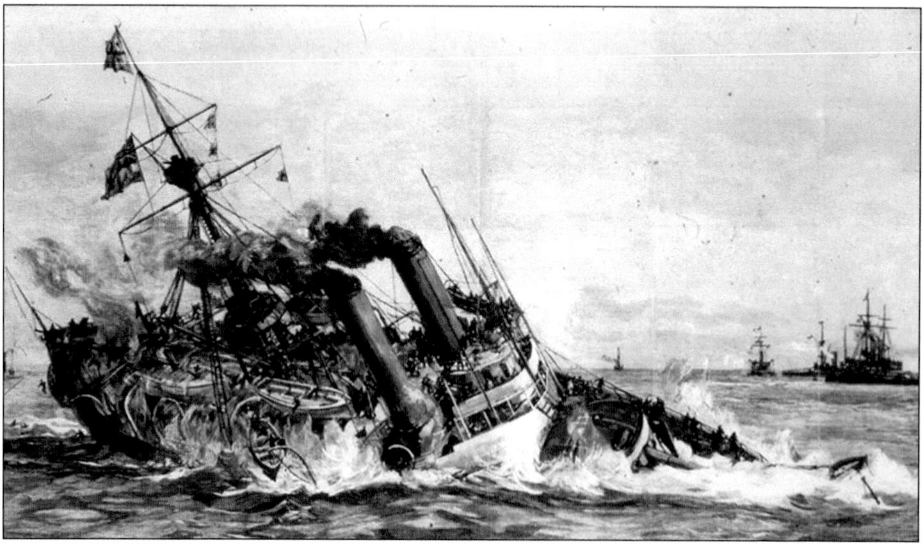

The loss of HMS *Victoria*, 22 June 1893. (Reproduced from *The Graphic*, 8 July 1893, with permission from The British Library)

In attempting to explain the disaster, the highly respected Admiral Sir Geoffrey Phipps Hornby speculated that Tryon was suffering from Mediterranean Fever:

> We know Sir George had been suffering very lately from fever; and I happen to have had painful evidence of how virulent Mediterranean Fever has been in the last two years. I have no doubt he was so suffering, and gave his orders in complete forgetfulness.[15]

This allegation was firmly refuted by Tryon's Fleet Surgeon, Mr Herbert Ellis, at the court-martial in Malta.

But was Malta Fever the culprit after all, the real villain of the piece? The other main protagonist, Rear Admiral Albert Markham, commanding *Camperdown*, had in February been struck down with Malta Fever, only returning from a prolonged convalescence to rejoin the Fleet four weeks before the fatal collision. Is it possible that Markham's slow reaction and erroneous interpretation of Tryon's signal were due to the after-effects of Malta Fever?[16]

15 G. P. Hornby, 'The Loss of the Victoria' in *United Service Magazine*, August 1893; 128: pp.1109–1113.

16 D. J. Vassallo, 'The Centenary of the Sinking of the Mediterranean Fleet flagship, HMS *Victoria*. What was the role of Malta Fever?' in *Journal of the Royal Navy Medical Service*,79, (1993), pp.91–99.

Rightly or wrongly, in the perceived opinion of the time, the loss of the Royal Navy's mightiest battleship and its most famous officer became inextricably linked to the mysterious microbe of Malta Fever.

This drew worldwide attention to the havoc this illness was causing to the Mediterranean garrison, and it thereby played a catalytic role in the saga of brucellosis, ultimately leading to the setting up of the Mediterranean Fever Commission.

In the meantime, this controversy spurred Louis Hughes, overseeing the fever wards in Malta, to determine the mode of transmission. The prevailing opinion was that the cause was sewage pollution of subsoil by leakage from broken cesspits.

Hughes, Undulant Fever and Goat's Milk

In 1896, Louis Hughes and his wife caught Malta Fever and were invalided home to Wales. His prolonged convalescence gave him the opportunity to write up his research, published in 1897 in an important monograph entitled *Mediterranean, Malta or Undulant Fever.*[17] Completed when Hughes was only 30 years old, this book firmly established his reputation.

Hughes coined the term 'undulant fever' because of the undulating character of the temperature, and because he disapproved of a limiting geographical term like 'Malta Fever'.

It was Bruce who had originally described the tendency of the fever to assume an 'undulatory course'. Ironically, Bruce hated the name given by Hughes, 'We trust that such a ridiculous term as 'undulant fever' will never come into general use.'[18]

However, in one important respect, Hughes went badly astray: he completely ruled out the possibility of milk being the vehicle of infection. He had 'met with no fact that would favour a causal connection between milk supply and this fever.'[19]

Ironically, Hughes came tantalisingly close to the solution, but failed to make the vital connection, in fact advocating goats' milk as treatment:

> In the countries where this fever occurs, **goats' milk is always obtainable**, cows' milk being less commonly used. As goats can generally be brought to the patient's house, or to the hospital, and there milked under supervision, their milk is to be preferred to the more doubtful cows' milk… [author's emphasis][20]

17 M. L. Hughes, *Mediterranean, Malta or Undulant Fever,* (London: Macmillan, 1897).
18 D. Bruce, 'Malta Fever Part II (Editorial)' in *Journal of the Royal Army Medical Corps*, June 1904, pp.731–736.
19 Hughes, *Mediterranean, Malta or Undulant Fever*, p.52.
20 Hughes, *Mediterranean, Malta or Undulant Fever*, p.91.

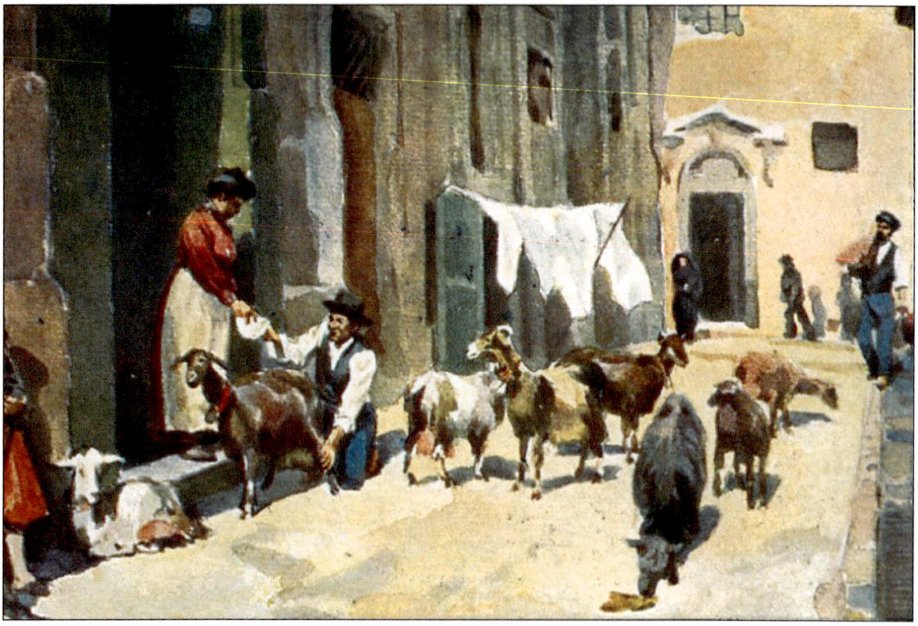

Maltese goatherd providing fresh milk. (Painting by Chevalier Edward Caruana Dingli, 1876-1950. Reproduced with permission of Perfecta Advertising Ltd)

His clearly documented case histories show that all his visiting relatives, his wife and himself fell severely ill with fever. The leaking drain in their backyard only reinforced his belief in the sewage theory.

One wonders whether Louis' enthusiasm for goats' milk may not have had a bearing on the severity and prolonged nature of their illness; his lasted 310 days:

> Milk, as fresh and pure as possible, should form the chief part of the patient's diet... As a general rule three pints of good milk is sufficient for a very severe case, every 24 hours. This may be increased in amount in less severe cases until a maximum of five pints is reached.[21]

One may imagine how meticulously Louis would have followed his own advice and served his nearest and dearest with five pints daily of fresh goats' milk obtained directly from their trusted milkman.

Despite the undoubted excellence of his book, Hughes' ideas on the place of milk in the management of Undulant Fever not only almost killed him and his stepsister, but they also delayed for years the discovery of how the disease was spread. No medical

21 Hughes, *Mediterranean, Malta or Undulant Fever*, p.190.

worker, after reading Hughes' authoritative statements, could possibly suspect the humble Maltese goat.

Louis Hughes died tragically, aged 32, at the Battle of Colenso on 15 December 1899 during the attempt to relieve the siege of Ladysmith in the Second Boer War. Coincidentally, only 15 miles north, besieged within Ladysmith itself, were David and Mary Bruce. Bruce was in charge of No.1 Stationary Hospital, running an improvised operating theatre, while Mary worked as his theatre sister. The newly created Royal Army Medical Corps (RAMC, formed 23 June 1898) was receiving its baptism of fire.

Laboratory diagnosis

Simultaneously with Hughes publishing his book, a major advance occurred in laboratory diagnosis. In 1897 Almroth Wright, Professor of Pathology at Netley, and Surgeon Major David Semple, Assistant Professor, successfully applied Widal's Agglutination Test to the testing of serum of Malta Fever patients, readily distinguishing it from typhoid fever, malaria and other illnesses.

The Widal test was promulgated in Malta by Caruana Scicluna and Zammit at the Public Health Department, though significantly their colleagues refused to use it. Local doctors were notoriously resistant to change and very suspicious of the public health authorities. They reacted similarly to Zammit's advocating the boiling of milk during an outbreak of gastroenteritis due to coliform contamination. The doctors objected on the grounds that 'To boil is to spoil.' Such ingrained beliefs bedevilled attempts to control Malta Fever.

Wright's modification of the Widal test was adopted by the British Army in Malta in 1900, and then by the Navy. It soon confirmed the clinical impression that Undulant Fever prevailed far beyond the Mediterranean basin, though it was not until 1902 that reliable statistics could be collected. In 1905 Zammit would apply this test to goats' milk, when it became known as Zammit's test.

Malaria and Malta

1897 was to be remembered for another momentous discovery: a surgeon with the Indian Army Medical Service, Ronald Ross, discovered malaria parasites in mosquitoes. Zammit enthusiastically corresponded with Ross, wondering whether Malta Fever might also be transmitted by mosquitoes. Zammit carried out extensive fieldwork without finding the Micrococcus, but in 1902 still contended that Malta Fever might be transmitted by insects.

The Origins of the Mediterranean Fever Commission

When David Bruce returned to England from South Africa, Zammit appraised him of his suspicions regarding mosquitoes. Bruce, elected a Fellow of the Royal Society while besieged in Ladysmith, brought this to the attention of the Royal Society.

As a result of Bruce's intervention, Sir Michael Foster, Secretary of the Royal Society, wrote on 2 December 1902 to the Under Secretary of State for the Colonies, requesting the Government's intercession with the Government of Malta on behalf of Dr Zammit. He advocated the creation of a formal investigation, to examine the possibility 'that Malta Fever is conveyed by means of a mosquito or other insect.'

The British Government, no longer distracted by war in South Africa, was increasingly concerned at the cost entailed by the equivalent of a regiment of infantry being ill at any one time with Malta Fever. The Royal Society's timely involvement culminated in the formation of the Mediterranean Fever Commission on 16 May 1904.

Bruce, Malta Fever and the Journal of the RAMC

It is pertinent to explore the relationship between Bruce, Malta Fever and the new *Journal of the RAMC* (hereafter *The Journal*), and to examine this journal's role as an all-important propaganda weapon in the war against this disease.

The Journal was founded in 1903, soon after the call from the Royal Society to investigate Malta Fever. Bruce, arguably the most famous officer in the newly created RAMC, was appointed editor in early 1904. He forthrightly converted *The Journal* into the mouthpiece through which each stage of the epic fight against this illness was broadcast to the world, commencing with his extensive editorial of April 1904 devoted to Malta Fever.[22]

He thundered out a challenge to the Government and the RAMC, 'There can be little doubt that it is in the investigation of disease with a view to its prevention that our foremost duty lies.'[23]

His April editorial carried blueprints for the necessary experiments. He would follow these almost to the letter when his efforts were rewarded by his appointment as Chairman of the Advisory Committee of the Royal Society supervising the MFC, on 16 May 1904. Subsequently, *The Journal* under his editorship would reprint all seven volumes of MFC Reports, ensuring their widest possible distribution, and their ready availability even today.

22 David Bruce, 'Malta Fever. Editorial' in *Journal of the Royal Army Medical Corps*, 2, (1904), pp.485–502.

23 David Bruce. 'Malta Fever. Editorial' in *Journal of the Royal Army Medical Corps* 2, (1904), pp.603–605.

The Mediterranean Fever Commission

The working members represented the Army, the Navy and the Civil Government, and initially consisted of Colonel David Bruce RAMC as president, Major William Heaton Horrocks, sanitary officer from Gibraltar, Staff Surgeon Ernest Shaw RN from HMS *Vulcan*, and Dr Temi Zammit, Board of Health, Malta. They were joined on 30 June by Dr Ralph Johnstone, an epidemiologist on loan from the Local Government Board.

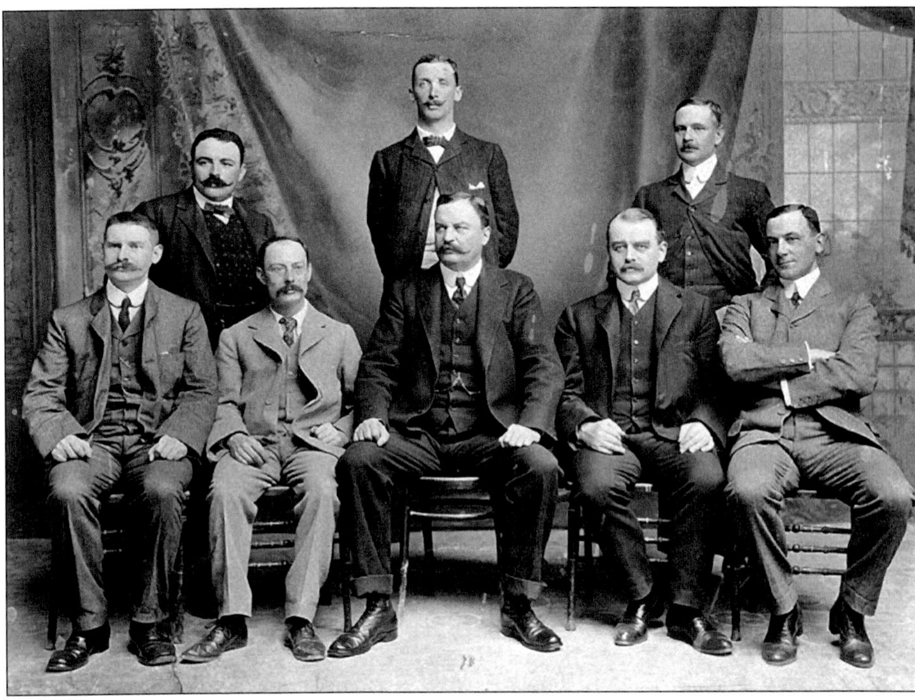

Mediterranean Fever Commission, 1904. (RAMC Muniments Collection, Wellcome Library. Copyrighted work available under Creative Commons by-nc 2.0 UK)

Late in 1904 they were joined by Captain James Crawford Kennedy RAMC (in charge of the Acute Fever Wards at the Station Hospital), and by Staff Surgeon Gilmour RN (Bighi Hospital). Later members included Lieutenant Colonel A. M. Davies RAMC, Dr J. W. H. Eyre (Bacteriologist to Guy's Hospital), Majors J. G. McNaught, T. McCulloch and J. C. Weir RAMC, Staff Surgeon F. H. A. Clayton RN, and Fleet Surgeon P. W. Bassett-Smith RN.

Bruce chose the Board of Health rooftop laboratory in Castellania Palace, Valletta, as the best location for the Commission. A plaque within this Palace (now the Ministry of Health) commemorates this association.[24] The roof was utilised for experiments on monkeys. Bruce returned to England in mid-July.

The first discovery of significance was made by Horrocks. He isolated the organism in the urine of infected patients, notifying Bruce by telegram on 22 July 1904. Soon another discovery was heralded. One can sense the suppressed excitement in Zammit's first letter to Bruce on 26 August:

> Today I find that one of my monkeys has developed a temperature, and has a blood reaction up to 1 in 300. The monkey had been bitten by two [mosquitoes] which had fed two days previously on a patient affected with Mediterranean Fever at the Civil Hospital.[25]

Zammit felt he was on the brink of an epochal discovery to rival that of Ross. Horrocks now started working on mosquitoes, writing to Bruce on 5 September: 'If I can confirm Zammit's results I think the work may be considered practically finished .... It seems to me the story is now pretty plain.'

However, the enigma was not to be solved so easily. On 23 September Horrocks reported: 'All the mosquito experiments have failed.'

Monkey Shortage

By far the greatest difficulty for the Commission was finding monkeys for experiments. They had to be imported at great expense from Calcutta and Ceylon, with consignments arriving irregularly and depleted by monkeys dying en route. It was also unfortunate that their chosen species, *Macacus Rhesus*, proved relatively resistant to infection, leading to erroneous conclusions when extrapolating results to man.

The monkeys were housed individually in cramped cages. In early September, two monkeys accidentally developed Mediterranean Fever, apparently from their immediate neighbours, causing Horrocks to write: 'These two results will invalidate monkey experiments on the terrace for some time to come.'[26] Horrocks had to kill off the infected monkeys, disinfect the roof, and segregate the few remaining monkeys.

24 Paul Cassar, *Sir Temi Zammit's Laboratory* (Malta: Department of Information, 1980).

25 The author's father obtained this and other quotes taken from correspondence between the members of the Mediterranean Fever Commission, from photocopies supplied by the Royal Society in the 1960s or early 70s. This correspondence is now held at the Wellcome Library (within the Contemporary Medical Archives Collection, CMAC WT1/RST files). For simplicity, quotations from these Letters are simply referenced by date and author in the body of this article.

26 Letter; Horrocks to Bruce, 8 September 1904.

Zammit's choice of Maltese Goats

Constrained to experimenting on the few monkeys at the Station Hospital, and encouraged by coincidentally discovering malaria transmission by mosquitoes in Malta on 13 September, Zammit looked for an alternative. His attention turned to the ubiquitous Maltese goat.

He obtained a goat on 15 September, confirmed that its blood reacted negatively for agglutinins, and commenced feeding experiments, buying another goat in December. Over subsequent months, he intermittently examined their blood, milk and urine, but was distracted by other duties. He was a gifted amateur archaeologist and was setting up the Malta Museum, which would be inaugurated on 25 May 1905. He was also lecturing in chemistry at the University of Malta and had applied for the Professorial post, being appointed in June 1905.

Nonetheless, during the winter of 1904/1905, realisation slowly dawned. While his two goats remained well, their serum converted from negative to a persistently positive reaction, leading Zammit to revise his previous belief in mosquito transmission of Malta Fever. By the time of the last positive agglutination test on 29 April he had formulated a new hypothesis: 'These two experiments led me to the belief that goats are susceptible to Malta Fever, and that the disease may be spread to human beings by goats.'[27]

Zammit would probably not have paid attention to goats had the supply of monkeys been plentiful. He waited until Bruce arrived in Malta (28 May 1905) so that he could personally communicate his serendipitous findings. This was the tipping point for the Commission. Bruce recorded this important meeting for posterity: 'Zammit informed the Chairman that the goat was in his opinion the transmitter of the disease...'[28]

Bruce's spirits must truly have been raised by this promising news, for only two weeks beforehand Staff Surgeon Shaw in Bighi Hospital had informed him that the Admiralty had ordered him to cease all animal experiments on Navy property, fearing the strong Anti-Vivisection movement in London.

Bruce was galvanised, as is evident from the MFC's records. The position at the beginning of June 1905 and the start of the new fever season looked much more promising. It remained to be seen if Zammit's new hypothesis could be proven.

27 T. Zammit. A Preliminary Note on the Susceptibility of Goats to Malta Fever. *Proceedings of the Royal Society*, 76B, (1905), pp.377–378. (Reprinted in: *Journal of the Royal Army Medical Corps*, 5, (1905), pp.341–342).

28 D. Bruce. Introduction. *Reports of Mediterranean Fever Commission*, Part III (London: Harrison & Sons, 1905), August: pp.3–4.

The Goats' Milk Discovery

Bruce left Malta on 12 June 1905. On the same day Zammit bought six goats from two different herds and took them to the Lazzaretto. On 14 June, he examined their blood. With mounting excitement, he discovered that the blood in five out of the six goats reacted strongly to the *Micrococcus Melitensis* in the specific agglutination test, indicating that they were naturally infected. He obtained identical results the next day. Horrocks and Shaw confirmed Zammit's findings.

At Caruana Scicluna's suggestion, Zammit had brought milk from each goat for examination. It was agreed that Zammit would investigate the bloods, and Horrocks the milk. Zammit reported the findings to Bruce by letter on 30 June:

> for the lazaretto I found that not less than five reacted to M.M. I informed Horrocks of the fact and passed him some milk for examination. He found the coccus in this milk and I found it abundant in the blood of the same goat. This is not bad for a beginning and hope to make good progress along the way.

Zammit sent his pithy, seminal report to the Royal Society, concluding that though the organism had caused no symptoms it must have lived and multiplied in the tissues.[29]

Controversy

The news of the discoveries of 14–15 June was first communicated to Bruce by Horrocks as Acting Chairman, whose letter of 20 June, intentionally or not, made it appear that the main credit was due to himself. Bruce was certainly given this impression. It was only when he received letters from Zammit dated 30 June and from Shaw dated 5 July that he became aware of the facts.

Nonetheless, the chase was on and Bruce's hunting instincts were to go for the kill:

> I was much excited by your letter this morning.... If this discovery in regard to the milk turns out to be true, it ought to make all your fortunes, it will be one of the most remarkable discoveries of recent times, and if the goat is the only transmitter of the disease we will be able to cut all their throats and throw them into the sea and "Bust the fever."[30]

The Maltese goatherds soon divined his intentions: 'I am afraid there is a combination of the owners of the goats against us; they are getting very suspicious and refuse to allow the goats to be touched...'[31]

29 Zammit. A Preliminary Note on the Susceptibility of Goats to Malta Fever. pp.377–378.
30 Letter, Bruce to Davies, 28 June 1905.
31 Letter, Horrocks to Bruce, 5 July 1905.

Zammit sidestepped obstacles by successfully adapting the agglutination test for milk, enabling widespread testing in villages and towns. The milkmen were happy to sell goats' milk, a much easier process than bleeding their goats. The results corroborated Zammit's suspicions, revealing that up to half of the 20,000 goats in Malta were infected and that a tenth were excreting the organism in their milk.[32]

The Pied Piper

Just as victory seemed assured, there was another twist to this tale. Lieutenant Colonel A. M. Davies, replacing Johnstone as epidemiologist in 1905, threw the cold water of doubt on the newly perceived importance of goats' milk in the causation of Malta Fever. My father described him as the pied piper who would lead the Commission astray.

Davies was pre-occupied with the soldiers' insanitary and poorly-ventilated barracks, and indeed his recommendations led to a marked improvement. He would eventually become the Army's Professor of Hygiene.

Within three weeks of Horrocks' intimation to Bruce that 'There may be something in the goat question.' Davies had investigated the milk supply for the 2nd Battalion of the Essex Regiment (who had suffered considerably from Mediterranean Fever at Lower St Elmo), and the Royal Garrison Artillery (who had suffered only slightly at Upper St Elmo). The findings perplexed him:

> I can ascertain no series of facts pointing with any clearness to milk-transmission as an important mode of spread among troops or families. Practically all the troops drink either boiled or condensed milk and the great majority of families do the same...[33]

It would be many months before realisation dawned on Davies, 'with Maltese cooks, possessed of profound faith in the virtues of goats' milk, we cannot be certain that effective sterilisation had been carried out.'

It was not just the local doctors who believed 'To boil is to spoil'.

Distractions

By the end of August 1905, the expert opinion of Davies dismissing the goats' milk theory created so much doubt that the Commission was led to waste time investigating alternative hypotheses. Thus, the incidental finding in September of micrococci in the blood of a mosquito that had fed on an infected monkey resulted in

32 J. C. Kennedy, 'Notes from Malta' in *Journal of the Royal Army Medical Corps*, 5, (1905), p.44.
33 Letter, Davies to Director General, 17 September 1905.

Horrocks and Kennedy setting themselves the tedious, and ultimately fruitless, task of dissecting 1,000 mosquitoes. This occupied six weeks.

Zammit's contention that infected goats' milk might be the mode of transmission was hotly disputed by Royal Navy Surgeons Edward H. Ross (brother of Ronald Ross) and G. Murray Levick aboard the cruiser HMS *Lancaster*, investigating mosquitoes around the Mediterranean.[34] They claimed to have drunk such milk without coming to harm.[35] Edward Ross, as a sailor, could not see how the ordinary 'Jack Tar' could possibly catch Malta Fever other than from biting insects when in harbour: 'The British sailor does not, as a rule, when he goes ashore at night on the spree, drink MILK.'

Bruce was exasperated by these delays and distractions:

> Can't you fellows give us a "tip" as to how this fever is spread? I thought the milk was going to explain everything, but neither Davies, Horrocks or any of you seem to think much of the milk...[36]

S.S. *Joshua Nicholson*

A fortuitous epidemic of brucellosis aboard ship stemmed the tide of scepticism. The merchant vessel S.S. *Joshua Nicholson*, trading between Antwerp and Egypt, anchored in Malta for one day in August 1905 to take on board 65 Milch goats bound for Washington. En route back to Antwerp, many of the ship's crew drank fresh goats' milk, and within weeks several were struck down with Malta Fever.

The first intimation of this was published in early 1906 as a short letter to Bruce from Dr N. Armand Ruffer, Maritime Quarantine Officer in Egypt.[37] Further details soon followed and Bruce expounded on this epidemic in two editorials.[38] This was clear proof of the connection of Malta Fever in man with the Maltese goat.

Royal Naval Hospital Bighi

Further positive epidemiological evidence was forthcoming when Shaw showed that a third of the Malta Fever cases in the Mediterranean Fleet occurred among staff

34 E. H. Ross, Levick G. Murray, 'Experiments on the transmission of Mediterranean Fever' in *Journal of the Royal Army Medical Corps*, 5, (1905), pp.240–247. E. H. Ross, Levick G. Murray, 'Notes on some of the Blood-sucking insects of the Mediterranean littoral' in *Journal of the Royal Army Medical Corps*, 5, (1905), pp.385–390.

35 E.H. Ross, Levick G. Murray, 'Dissemination of Malta Fever by Goats' Milk. (Correspondence)' in *Journal of the Royal Army Medical Corps*, 5, (1905), p.662.

36 Letter, Bruce to Shaw, 25 January 1906.

37 Armand N. Ruffer, 'The possible infection of man with Micrococcus Melitensis by oats' milk. (Correspondence)' in *Journal of the Royal Army Medical Corps*, 6, (1906), p.113.

38 D. Bruce. Editorial. *Journal of the Royal Army Medical Corps*, 6, (1906), pp.65–167; D. Bruce. Malta Fever (Editorial). *Journal of the Royal Army Medical Corps*, 6, (1906), pp.330–352.

and patients at Bighi hospital. He discovered that the herds of goats supplying this hospital were heavily infected with the Micrococcus.[39]

Negative epidemiological evidence was also forthcoming. Dr Caruana Scicluna showed that none of the 200 inmates of an Institution run by nuns had suffered from Malta Fever for many years. Examination of the Institution's goats revealed them to be uninfected. Similarly, there had been no cases of Malta Fever in the overcrowded, insanitary Civil Prison for over nine years – this was ascribed to the prisoners not being allowed milk in any form.

Affirmative Action

Bruce returned to Malta in April 1906. With three new epidemiologists on the Commission, and all the accumulated evidence before him, Bruce could finally write categorically to the Lieutenant Governor on 1 May, two days before leaving Malta:

> In conclusion, I beg to record my opinion that the infection of man with Mediterranean Fever by means of goats' milk is one of the most important factors in the spread of this disease … and that I think the time has come when measures to remove this danger to the Public Health should forthwith be undertaken.

The Governor responded robustly with an Order to the Garrison on 12 May:

> Stop goats' milk to troops; interim arrangements: use condensed tinned milk…

The milkmen, their livelihood threatened, rose up in protest, pasting placards listing their grievances, signed 'The Vexed Maltese Milkman', and went on strike, between 15 and 30 May 1906. This resulted in the troops converting wholesale to tinned condensed milk. When the milkmen ended their strike, the troops would no longer buy their milk; their actions inadvertently made it easier for the military authorities to institute the necessary public health measures, reinforced by military discipline. This included the orders:

> *Goats' Milk prohibited by Army*' (Garrison Orders, June 1906)
> *Prohibition of use of unboiled goats' milk* (C-in-C's General Order to the Fleet, August 1906)

39 E.A. Shaw. III. 'Mediterranean Fever in goats, cows, and other animals. Reports of the MFC', 1906, Pt. IV, 16–26 (reprinted in: *Journal of the Royal Army Medical Corps*, 2, (1907),1). E.A. Shaw. III. Further Observations on goats, cats, rats, and ambulatory cases in connection with Mediterranean Fever. Reports of the MFC, 1906, Pt. V, 37–41.

Success at last

Bruce was able to appraise Sir Archibald Geikie FRS, Secretary of Royal Society, on 8 October 1906:

> Whether *post hoc* or *propter hoc*, it is too early to say, but during July, August and September of this year, there were only 15 cases of Malta Fever admitted to hospital against 258 cases for the corresponding three months of 1905 .... I think it is very probable that we have made a hit in preventive medicine, to the glory of God and the honour of our country...

Bruce had ended his May 1904 editorial with this exhortation:

> One thing appears perfectly clear, at least to our mind, and that is that no stone should be left unturned, no amount of labour thought too much, to enable us to gain a knowledge of the natural history of Malta Fever, and so in time to prevent the occurrence of so many cases of this plague among our soldiers and sailors in the Mediterranean.[40]

His efforts had been vindicated.

Bibliography

Manuscripts

RAMC Muniments Collection – Archives and manuscripts related to Sir David Bruce and Lady Bruce https://wellcomecollection.org/works/srscccsk (accessed 31 May 2024)

Books

Hughes, M. L., *Mediterranean, Malta or Undulant Fever* (London: Macmillan, 1897)

Journal articles

Anonymous, 'Obituary, Sir David Bruce' in *Obituary Notices of Fellows of the Royal Society*, 1 (1932), 79–85

Bruce, D., 'Note on the Discovery of a Micro-organism in Malta Fever' in *Practitioner*, 39 (1887) pp.161–170

Bruce, D., 'The Micrococcus of Malta Fever' in *Practitioner*, 40 (1888), pp.241–249

Bruce, D., 'Malta Fever. Editorial' in *Journal of the Royal Army Medical Corps*, 2 (1940), pp.485–502

40 D. Bruce. Malta Fever. Editorial, *Journal of the Royal Army Medical Corps*, 2, (1904), pp.603–605.

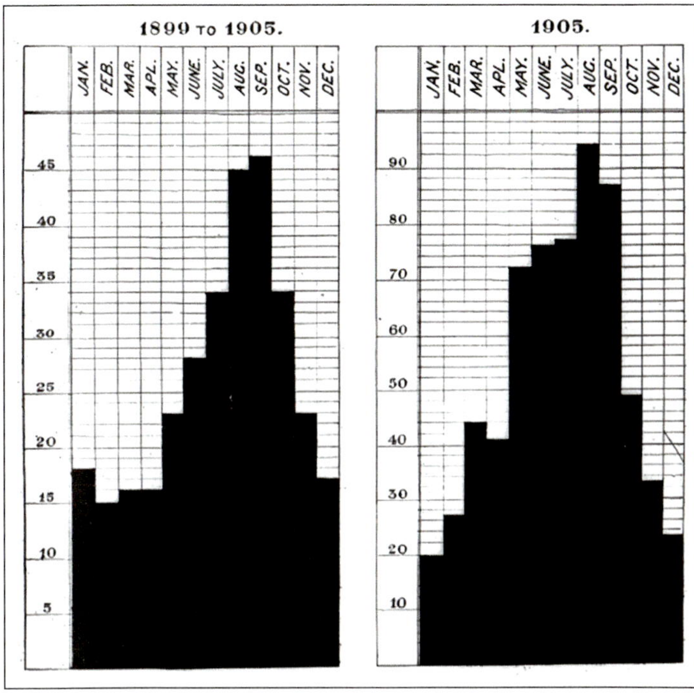

Prevalence of Malta Fever in the Garrison, 1899–1905. (Chart by David Bruce, RAMC Muniments Collection, Wellcome Library)

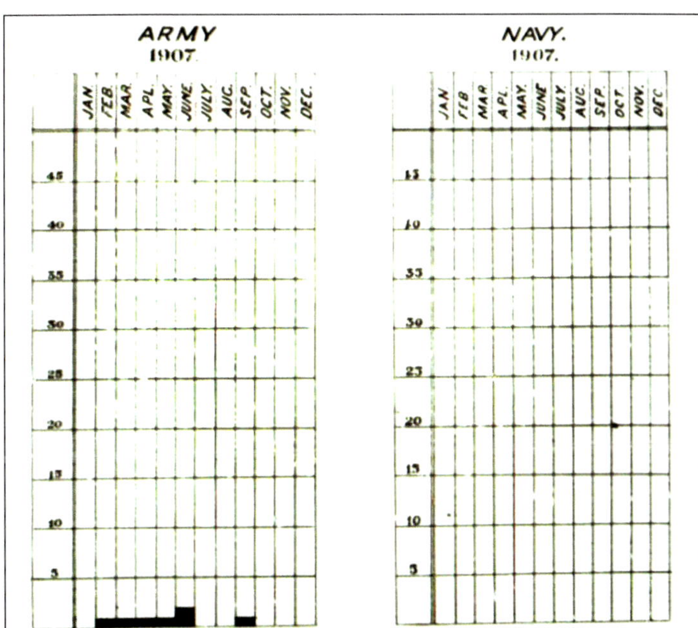

Prevalence of Malta Fever in the Garrison, 1907. (Chart by David Bruce, RAMC Muniments Collection, Wellcome Library)

Bruce, D., 'Malta Fever. Editorial' in *Journal of the Royal Army Medical Corps,* 2 (1904) pp.603–605
Bruce D. 'Malta Fever Part II. Editorial' in *Journal of the Royal Army Medical Corps*, 2 (1904), pp.731–736
Bruce, D., Editorial. *Journal of the Royal Army Medical Corps,* 6 (1906), pp.165–167
Bruce, D., 'Malta Fever' (Editorial) in *Journal of the Royal Army Medical Corps,* 6 (1906), pp.330–352
Hamerton, A. E., 'Obituary, Major-General Sir David Bruce' in *Transactions of the Royal Society of Tropical Medicine and Hygiene*, 25 (1931–1932), pp.305–312
Hornby, G. P., 'The Loss of the Victoria' in *United Service Magazine*, August 1893, 128, pp.1109–1113
Hughes, G. W. G., Hughes, M. H., 'Matthew Louis Hughes and Undulant Fever' in *Journal of the Royal Army Medical Corps* 115 (1969), pp.199–203
Kennedy, J. C., 'Notes from Malta' in *Journal of the Royal Army Medical Corps,* 5 (1905), p.44
Marston, J. A., 'Report on Fever (Malta)' in *Army Medical Department Medical Report for 1861,* 3 (1863), pp.520–521
Noble, J. E., 'The David Bruce Laboratories 25th anniversary' in *Journal of the Royal Army Medical Corps* 113 (1967), pp.208–212
Ross E. H., Murray Levick G., 'Experiments on the transmission of Mediterranean Fever' in *Journal of the Royal Army Medical Corps* 5 (1905), pp.240–247
Ross E. H., Murray, Levick G., 'Notes on some of the Blood-sucking insects of the Mediterranean littoral' in *Journal of the Royal Army Medical Corps,* 5 (1905), pp.85–390
Ross, E. H., Murray Levick G., 'Dissemination of Malta Fever by Goats' Milk' in *Journal of the Royal Army Medical Corps,* 5 (1905), p.62
Ruffer, Armand N., 'The Possible Infection of Man with Micrococcus Melitensis by Goats' Milk' in *Journal of the Royal Army Medical Corps*, 6 (1906), p.113
Vassallo, D. J., 'The Centenary of the Sinking of the Mediterranean Fleet Flagship, HMS *Victoria*. What was the role of Malta Fever?' in *Journal of the Royal Navy Medical Service,* 79 (1993), pp.91–99
Vassallo D. J., 'L. A. Vassallo, (Obituary)' in *British Medical Journal,* 309 (1994), p.1578
Vassallo D. J., The Saga of Brucellosis: controversy over credit for linking Malta Fever with goats' milk' in *The Lancet* 348 (1996), pp.804–808
Vella, E. E., 'Major-General Sir David Bruce, K.C.B.' in *Journal of the Royal Army Medical Corps* 119 (3) (1973), pp.131–144
Zammit, T. A., 'Preliminary Note on the Susceptibility of Goats to Malta Fever' in *Proceedings of the Royal Society,* 76B (1905), pp.377–378. Reprinted in: *Journal of the Royal Army Medical Corps* 5 (1905), pp.341–342

Publications

Cassar, Paul, *Sir Temi Zammit's Laboratory* (Malta: Department of Information, 1980)

Reports

Bruce, D., Introduction. Reports of Mediterranean Fever Commission, Part III (London: Harrison & Sons, 1905 August 3–4)

Shaw, E. A. III, 'Mediterranean Fever in goats, cows, and other animals.' Reports of the MFC 1906, Pt. IV, 16–26 (reprinted in: *Journal of the Royal Army Medical Corps*, 2 (1907), pp.1–12)

Shaw, E. A. III, 'Further Observations on goats, cats, rats, and ambulatory cases in connection with Mediterranean Fever' Reports of the MFC, 1906, Pt. V, 37–41.

Lectures

Bruce, David, Lecture to medical students, Aberdeen University, 1922

11

The Scottish Women's Hospitals' Orthopaedic Centre, Salonika

Elaine Morrison and Carol Parry

During the First World War orthopaedic centres were established in the UK to deal with the large numbers of wounded men returning from the front. A similar centre, based on those in the UK, was established in Salonika (modern day Thessaloniki), by the Girton and Newnham Unit of the Scottish Women's Hospitals (SWH). This Chapter will outline why and how it was established and equipped, the treatments offered, and the challenges associated with a centre based so far away from the large orthopaedic hospitals in the UK.

The SWH was formed shortly after the outbreak of the First World War. Dr Elsie Inglis, an Edinburgh obstetrician and gynaecologist and Honorary Secretary of the Scottish Federation of Women's Suffrage Societies, offered medical assistance to the British War Office in the form of a voluntary hospital staffed by women. When rebuffed, units were offered instead to the Allied Forces and France, Serbia and Russia accepted the offer of help.

The Girton and Newnham Unit

The Girton and Newnham Unit was funded initially by donations from former students of the two Cambridge women's colleges and formed the Second French Unit of the SWH. The unit established a tented hospital in Troyes in May 1915, working directly with the French Army. In the autumn of 1915, the unit was selected to join the French Expeditionary Force to Serbia. The Allied Forces arrived too late to save Serbia and the unit joined the general retreat to Salonika and established a hospital at Kalamaria, on the outskirts of the city.[1]

1 Elaine Morrison and Carol Parry, 'The Girton and Newnham Unit of the Scottish Women's Hospitals During the First World War' in *Journal of the Royal College of Physicians*, 44:4 (London: 2014), pp.337–343.

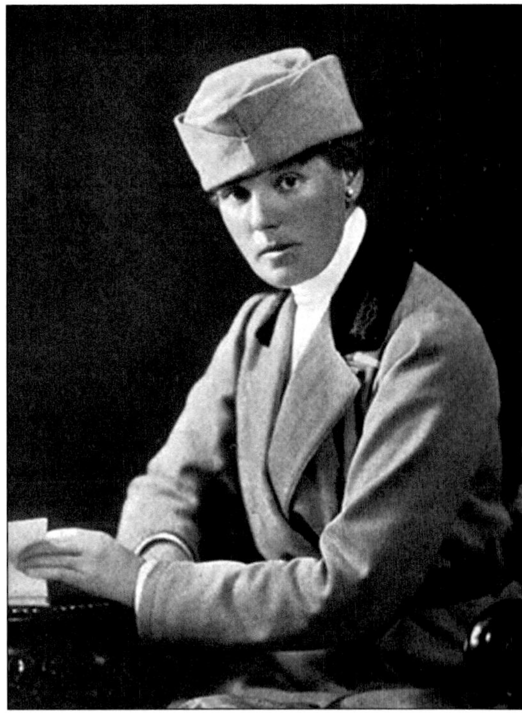

Dr (later Dame) Louise McIlroy, Chief Medical Officer of the Girton and Newnham Unit. (Photograph courtesy Glasgow City Archives)

In the course of her work there, Glasgow graduate Dr Louise McIlroy, the unit's Chief Medical Officer (CMO), became very interested in the rehabilitation of disabled soldiers. Wounded Serbs could not return home as their country was occupied by enemy forces and, given the distances and dangers involved in transporting men of the Allied Forces back home, it was quickly realised that rehabilitation facilities were required locally. In this, Louise McIlroy was greatly aided by Edith Stoney, a former Newnham College student and lecturer in physics at the London School of Medicine for Women, who ran the unit's X-ray department and was also its electrician. Edith Stoney had knowledge and experience in the use of various electrotherapies and had brought out electrical massage equipment with her from the UK. In addition, she had purchased a high-frequency therapy unit in Paris before leaving for Salonika. Rudimentary hot-air baths were constructed from old petrol cans by her assistant, George Mallett (one of the few men in the unit), and an old cocoa tin was used as a shade for a hot lamp. Stoney and Mallet were also able to create basic mechano-therapeutic equipment, later supplemented by bicycle wheels and bars sent out from the UK. Louise McIlroy realised that this treatment was 'one of the most important of the war for softening stiff joints.'[2]

Patients from other French hospitals were sent for treatment as well as several British officers, including the British Fleet's Surgeon General.[3] Despite the work being done in the Command Depots and Convalescent Camps in the UK at this

2 Glasgow City Archives TD1734/2/3/2/1(1/4) Letter from Louise McIlroy to Miss May, 20 September 1916; Adrian Thomas, Francis Duck, *Edith and Florence Stoney, Sisters in Radiology* (Cham, Switzerland: Springer, 2019), pp.195–205.

3 TD1734/9/1/2/24 Letter of Edith Stoney, 25 February 1916.

time, the RAMC were slow in using such methods in the field.[4] Dr Wilfrid Garton, radiologist to the 49th General Hospital, brought out his own galvanic battery but no other RAMC hospital in Salonika had electro-therapy facilities at that time.[5]

Establishing an orthopaedic centre

The initial electrical and mechano-therapeutic work carried out by the unit proved the utility of establishing a proper orthopaedic centre. However, they were hampered by the lack of space at Kalamaria and its low-lying site which was prone to flooding. These difficulties, though, did not stop Louise McIlroy from outlining her plans for further orthopaedic work to the SWH Hospitals Committee in Edinburgh:

> I want to get a department as soon as I can get more ground space and tents. We have had some awfully good results from our cases here I want to go on and develop the whole thing.[6]

She realised that much had moved on in the field of orthopaedics since she left Scotland and had heard of centres such as Bellahouston near Glasgow, and Bangour near Edinburgh, both based on the ideas of the RAMC's Director of Military Orthopaedics, Sir Robert Jones.

The model for such centres was the Military Orthopaedic Hospital, Shepherd's Bush, opened in March 1916 with Jones guiding the establishment of further centres throughout the UK.[7] In addition to its surgical department, the centre at Shepherd's Bush provided electrical treatment, massage, hydrotherapy, physical activities in a gymnasium and curative workshops. The latter had been introduced by King Manoel of Portugal, a member of the Joint War Committee of the Red Cross and Order of St John, and were based on those at the Anglo-Belgian Hospital in Rouen and the Canadian Hospital in Ramsgate. The curative workshops were felt to be beneficial physically and psychologically; providing a means of exercising limbs as well as offering something useful to do, such as learning a new skill.[8]

At the request of Louise McIlroy, members of the Committee visited the Scottish National Red Cross Hospital at Bellahouston, Glasgow, but concluded that it would be impossible 'to undertake such work on the present site' at Kalamaria.[9] In the

4 See F.B. Lambert, 'Massage and Medical Electricity in the After-Treatment of Convalescent Soldiers' in *The Lancet,* 4 November 1916 (London: 1916), pp.788–790.
5 Letter of Wilfrid Garton, 'Electrotherapeutics in Military Hospitals' in *British Medical Journal,* 16 September 1939 (London: 1939), p.622.
6 TD1734/2/3/2/1 (1/4) Letter from Louise McIlroy to Miss May, 20 September 1916.
7 Roger Cooter, *Surgery and Society in Peace and War: Orthopaedics and the Organisation of Modern Medicine, 1880–1948* (Basingstoke: Macmillan, 1993), pp.105–106.
8 Cooter, p.118.
9 TD1734/1/2/1/6 Hospitals Committee minutes, 8 August 1917.

meantime, Edith Stoney's small electrical department continued to provide excellent results, Louise McIlroy writing in June 1917 that:

> A short time ago I received a visit from an officer on the staff of a very well-known General out here saying he (the General) had been suffering from severe neuralgia in his arm and side, and that, on consulting the British medical general he said "We cannot give you the proper electrical treatment. You must go down to the Scottish Women. They are the only people who can treat you out here." He is having applications (as an outpatient) of hot air, light, high frequency and massage, and is greatly benefitted by it and is spreading our fame all over the place.[10]

At long last, in August 1917, the French agreed to move the unit to a more suitable new site, increasing the number of beds from 300 to 500. The new site, located on a hillside outside Salonika was spacious with good drainage and an adequate water supply. Wasting no time, Louise McIlroy returned to Scotland in September on a fact-finding holiday, leaving the unit's Administrator, Lillian Laloë to organise the move. Louise McIlroy attended a meeting of the Committee in Edinburgh on 19 September and asked for permission to commence orthopaedic work, stating that she planned to visit orthopaedic departments in Scotland and England to see all the latest developments. Following the meeting, the Committee decided that money raised by Mrs Elizabeth Abbott in India, via the Caledonian Society of Calcutta, should be used to 'establish, maintain and equip' the proposed orthopaedic department in Salonika and that it would be called the 'Calcutta Orthopaedic Centre'.[11]

Inspiration from British centres

Louise McIlroy first visited Bangour, a former psychiatric hospital outside Edinburgh, which had been requisitioned by the War Office. Bangour had 500 beds set aside for orthopaedic patients and a large hydrotherapeutic department was in the process of being built. By the time of her visit, the electrical department was well established under Thomas Rankine and was said to be 'exceptionally good'.[12] Her next two visits were to hospitals closer to her home in Glasgow. The orthopaedic department at Bellahouston, housed in a new building, provided the latest physical and mechanical forms of treatment, including hydrotherapy. There were 'separate rooms for heat in the form of baths, for massage, remedial exercises, for electricity, and also for radiant heat.' The whirlpool and pool baths furnished 'air and water in rapid motion and at high temperatures, their main object being

10 TD1734/9/1/2/20 Louise McIlroy to Miss May, 5 June 1917.
11 TD1734/1/2/1/6 Hospitals Committee minutes, 19 September 1917.
12 Anonymous, 'Curative Workshops' in *British Medical Journal*, 5 May 1917, (London: 1917), pp.585–586.

to prepare an affected limb or part for massage, for manipulation, and for movement of the joints or muscles.'[13] More than 100 men were working in the curative workshops.

Not far from Glasgow, along the banks of the Clyde, was the Princess Louise Hospital situated at Erskine, founded at the instigation of Glasgow surgeon, Sir William Macewen. The hospital had begun admitting patients in October 1916 and specialised in the aftercare of amputation cases with workshops for amputees. Like the centre at Shepherd's Bush, inspiration for these had come from the Anglo-Belgian Hospital at Rouen.[14] Macewen was determined that artificial limbs should be manufactured at the hospital with input from the patients. Local Glasgow shipyards, particularly Yarrow's, offered their help in the manufacture and design of limbs. Thus, Louise McIlroy was able to see artificial limbs being made which was helpful in deciding whether this would be feasible in Salonika. She also visited Messrs Shanks of Barrhead. In addition to general sanitary ware, the company had become prominent in the supply and manufacture of therapeutic baths for hydrotherapy.[15]

Louise McIlroy then travelled south to visit orthopaedic centres in England. A special meeting of the Committee was held in Edinburgh on 27 October to hear the results of her investigations. At the meeting McIlroy reported that she had visited the best orthopaedic hospitals in Scotland and England and spoken with specialists in the field. She was able to lay before the Committee estimates for a whole bath department from Shanks which included all types of baths currently in use in similar departments and a hut to house them. She also had estimates for an electrical outfit from Messrs Trotter of Glasgow who had supplied the apparatus at Bellahouston Hospital and for gymnastic apparatus from Spencer, Heath & George Ltd, London, a firm specialising in mechanical apparatus for post-surgical treatment of the wounded. The apparatus included pulley weight machines, a nautical wheel, an exercise bicycle, dumbbells, Indian clubs, a rowing machine and six massage tables.[16]

Based on the knowledge gained on her tour of orthopaedic centres, Louise McIlroy suggested workshops for carpentry, iron work, leather work, tailoring and one for making stumps for amputees. These too, had all been costed, with the choice of tools and suppliers based on her visits. She realised that making artificial limbs would be too difficult, but it would be possible to create temporary stumps to enable amputees to walk about. By 12 December 1917, all the orders for the orthopaedic department had been given, at a total cost of around £5,000.[17]

13 Anonymous, 'Bellahouston Red Cross Hospital: New Orthopaedic Department' in *Glasgow Medical Journal*, 87:1, 1917 (Glasgow:1917), pp.41–43.
14 Jennifer Novotny, 'To "take their place among the productive members of society": Vocational rehabilitation of WWI wounded at Erskine', *Wellcome Open Research*, 2:5 (London: 2017), pp.1–9, 4.
15 F. P. Nunneley, 'The Whirlpool Bath' in *British Medical Journal*, 25 November 1916 (London:1916), pp.721–722.
16 TD1734/6/3/1/5 (2/2) Invoice from Spencer, Heath & George Ltd, London, 28 December 1917.
17 TD1734/1/2/1/6 Hospitals Committee minutes, 19 September 1917–14 November 1917.

In addition to her visits to orthopaedic centres in the UK, Louise McIlroy took the opportunity on her way back to Salonika to visit St Maurice, a hospital near Paris, where artificial limbs were manufactured under the auspices of the American Red Cross. However, having visited all these centres she felt that the methods used in Scotland were 'well to the fore' and it was certainly Bellahouston, Erskine and Bangour that informed her choices when it came to equipment.[18]

The Calcutta Orthopaedic Centre

The Calcutta Orthopaedic Centre was based in one of the huts that the French Army had given to the unit when it moved to its new site. Massage formed a major part of the treatment regimen and trained masseuses were recruited from orthopaedic centres in the UK, the number working at the hospital rising from one in March 1918 to eight in February 1919. The Incorporated Society of Trained Masseuses (ISTM) was founded in 1900 and the masseuse (the forerunner of today's physiotherapist) had already become an established occupation for women before the outbreak of the First World War. Demand for this work grew as the war progressed and new training schools were established offering ISTM qualifications. Virtually all the masseuses recruited for the unit obtained their qualifications during the war. They were hard-working and thrilled with their new equipment, starting work at 6.00 am during the summer to avoid the relentless heat of the Macedonian sun. Just like the centres in the UK they provided massage, electrical Faradic treatment and exercise classes. Several of the masseuses had certificates in medical electricity and two of the first three appointed had received special training in 'physical culture'.[19] Orthopaedic patients were sent from other French hospitals and Serbian depots and stayed in the hospital for around six months on average, so once all the beds were taken there was little opportunity to take in large numbers of new cases.[20] As the need for treatment was far greater than the number of beds available, some patients attended on an outpatient basis but it was difficult for them to receive continuous treatment because of transport difficulties.[21] In addition to the masseuses, the unit was loaned a Drill Sergeant from the British Army. This proved to be a great success: 'the patients are so happy with their drill and games'.[22]

Edith Stoney left the unit for a much-needed break in August 1917 with every intention of returning to Salonika. However, she was sent instead to the SWH's unit at Royaumont, near Paris. This was a severe blow. In April 1918, Louise McIlroy wrote to the Committee: 'What about a radiologist? I am in despair .... orthopaedic work will

18 TD1734/2/3/1/3 (3/3) Letter from Louise McIlroy to Miss May, 20 December 1917.
19 TD1734/1/4/3 Personnel Committee minutes, 19 February 1918.
20 TD1734/9/1/1/19 Letter from Louise McIlroy to Miss Ferguson, 9 October 1918.
21 TD1734/9/1/1/19 Letter from Louise McIlroy to Miss Ferguson, 28 January 1919.
22 TD1734/2/3/1/5 (2/3) Letter from Miss Laloë to Miss Ferguson, 5 March 1919.

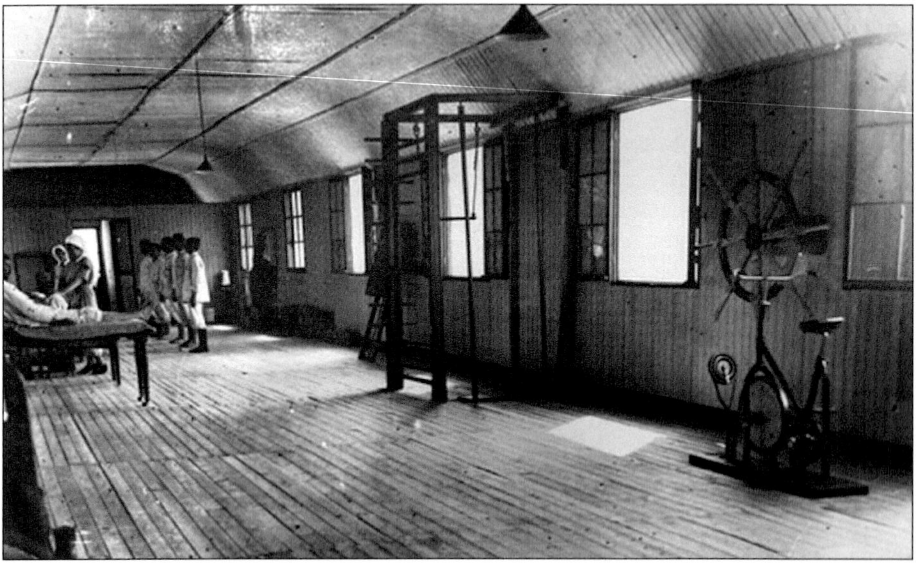

The Calcutta Orthopaedic Centre, Salonika. (Image courtesy of Glasgow City Archives)

be at a stand-still until one arrives.'[23] The following month the Committee managed to appoint Barbara Stephen as Assistant Radiographer. Although she was by no means as versatile or as knowledgeable as Edith Stoney, X-ray work could begin again.

Establishing an orthopaedic centre far away from the UK was ambitious and not without many problems. Items sent out from home took a long time to arrive, sometimes getting lost during the voyage or falling foul of new export regulations. Help was sought from senior members of the British Army in Salonika. Brigadier General Charles Fortescue, the British representative of the Serbian Joint Supply Commission, offered to help the unit to obtain supplies more quickly via the British Army and sent a wire to the War Office to get the hydrotherapeutic hut and equipment sent out as quickly as possible.[24] His wire had little effect as the hut and equipment did not arrive until the unit was in the process of moving to Serbia in early 1919 and had to be sent on to Belgrade. The mechano-therapeutic equipment arrived in April 1918, but without any assembly instructions (apart from the rowing machine). Nevertheless, the staff managed to assemble everything without them. The electrical equipment took longer to arrive. The electric light baths did not arrive until the end of July, and the staff just had to make the best of it: 'How one envies the home hospitals with all their experts,' wrote Louise McIlroy.[25] Even the beds that had been ordered as part of the enlargement of the hospital in November 1917 only started arriving in stages almost a

23 TD1734/2/3/2/8 (1/2) Letter from Louise McIlroy to Miss Kemp, 14 April 1918.
24 TD1734/2/3/2/8 (1/2) Letter from Louise McIlroy to Miss Kemp, 14 April 1918.
25 TD1734/2/3/2/8 (1/2) Letter from Louise McIlroy to Miss Kemp, 22 May 1918.

year later. In addition, having an orthopaedic centre so near to the front line and part of a general hospital also meant that, as the fighting on the front heated up during the summer of 1918, some orthopaedic beds had to be cleared for casualties.

Despite the difficulties, workshops under canvas were quickly established almost as soon as the hospital reopened for patients in the spring of 1918. A carpenters' workshop was set up to help in the building and equipping of the hospital supplying tables, chairs and doors, et cetera. Shoemakers mended the shoes of patients and staff and were also taught to make orthopaedic boots with cork obtained from a wine shop in Salonika.[26] A cigarette-making class was started for soldiers with disabled hands – tobacco and paper for rolling into a cigarette was given in exchange for 20 dead flies.[27] Some of the men were taught embroidery, copying Macedonian and Egyptian designs and these were then later sold to raise money for the workshops. Louise McIlroy was thrilled with the results: 'It is very wonderful what our men have done, working with mutilated hands and they are men who have been perhaps only labourers before the war.'[28] The unit's orderlies supervised the workshops but craftsmen to teach the men were in very short supply and the temporary limbs made out of pegs and plaster were far from adequate, the Serbian soldiers wanting to 'have one made of leather and hinges with a proper hand and foot.'[29] Malaria was an ever-present problem: 'The work is somewhat difficult as so often a good patient is stopped for days owing to an attack of malaria. It is the curse of regular work out here.'[30]

By the end of 1918 Louise McIlroy was able to report that since May of that year 426 patients had been treated, with 17,823 massage treatments and 2,543 Faradic treatments. With the Centre so much in demand, Louise McIlroy wished that she had many more beds and double the number of masseuses, especially with the realisation that early intervention was important. Theirs was not, however, the only orthopaedic centre in Salonika. At almost the same time, the RAMC established an Orthopaedic Curative Depot (No. 5 Convalescent Camp), also using the methods utilised by Jones with a similar regimen of massage, exercises and curative work. Their curative workshops included brickmaking, gardening and a joiners' shop. There was also a splint factory which was able to produce Thomas's walking calliper splints and a simple artificial leg.[31] Louise McIlroy was well aware that the SWH might not be the only ones wanting to work in this field as the British had always been 'most interested' in what she was planning. She aimed high and 'would have liked to have done it for all.'[32] However, being the only orthopaedic centre in Salonika for Serbian and French soldiers was a not inconsiderable achievement.

26 TD1734/2/3/1/4 (3/3) Letter from Louise McIlroy to Miss Ferguson, 6 November 1918.
27 TD1734/2/3/1/4 (1/3) Letter from Louise McIlroy to Miss Ferguson, 10 June 1918.
28 TD1734/2/3/1/4 (3/3) Letter from Louise McIlroy to Miss Ferguson, 13 December 1918.
29 TD1734/2/3/1/5 (1/3) Letter from Louise McIlroy to Miss Ferguson, 22 January 1919.
30 TD1734/2/3/1/4 (3/3) Letter from Louise McIlroy to Miss Ferguson, 13 December 1918.
31 T. Crisp English & R. E. Kelly, 'Notes on Surgery at Salonica' in *British Medical Journal* (16 March 1918), pp.305–310, 309.
32 TD1734/9/1/2/20 Letter from Louise McIlroy to Miss May, 6 July 1917.

During the course of 1918, the Girton and Newham Unit welcomed many important visitors including King Alexander of Greece. However, perhaps the most important personally for the CMO, Dr Louise McIlroy, and a vindication of all the hard work, was a meeting of the British Army Medical Society hosted by the unit on 5 June 1918 with Sir Maurice Holt, the Director of Medical Services, in the chair. There was a great deal of interest in the hospital and its apparatus and over 70 members attended, including several French and Serbian medical officers. Louise McIlroy led the proceedings with a paper on the 'Treatment and Re-education of the disabled soldier'. Following the meeting Colonel Straitch, a physician at the Serbian Crown Prince Alexander's Hospital, sent Louise McIlroy a letter thanking her for 'the interest you personally pay to this very serious and important problem, as well as for the interest you have succeeded to raise in Allied military and governmental circles here for the same.'[33] A tremendous accolade indeed for the only female CMO serving with the Allied Forces in Salonika.

Bibliography

Archive Sources

Glasgow City Archives TD1734 Records of the Scottish Women's Hospitals for Foreign Service: TD1734/1/2/1/6 Hospitals Committee minutes, 1917–1919; TD1734/1/4/3 Personnel Committee minutes, 1917–1920; TD1734/2/3/1 Circulated letters (1st Series), 1915–1922; TD1734/2/3/2 Circulated letters (2nd Series), 1915–1918; TD1734/6/3/1/5 Supplies and Equipment, Vouchers and receipted bills, 1917–1918; TD1734/9/1/2/20 Individual Correspondence, Dr A. Louise McIlroy, 1915–1918; TD1734/9/1 2nd French Unit Correspondence, 1915–1921

Books

Cooter, Roger, *Surgery and Society in Peace and War: Orthopaedics and the Organisation of Modern Medicine, 1880–1948* (Basingstoke: Macmillan, 1993)

Thomas, Adrian and Duck, Francis, *Edith and Florence Stoney, Sisters in Radiology* (Cham, Switzerland: Springer, 2019)

Journal Articles

Anonymous, 'Bellahouston Red Cross Hospital: New Orthopaedic Department' in *Glasgow Medical Journal*, 87:1 (Glasgow: 1917), pp.41–43

Anonymous, 'Curative Workshops' in *British Medical Journal*, 5 May 1917 (London 1917), pp.585–586 English, T. Crisp and Kelly, R. E., 'Notes on Surgery at Salonica' in *British Medical Journal*, 16 March 1918 (London:1918), pp.305–310

33 TD1734/2/3/1/4 (1/3) Letter from Colonel Straitch to Louise McIlroy, 7 June 1918.

Garton, Wilfred, 'Electrotherapeutics in Military Hospitals' in *British Medical Journal*, 16 September 1939 (London: 1939), p.622

Lambert, F. B. 'Massage and Medical Electricity in the After-Treatment of Convalescent Soldiers' in *The Lancet*, 4 November 1916 (London: 1916), pp.788–90

Morrison, Elaine and Parry, Carol, 'The Girton and Newnham Unit of the Scottish Women's Hospitals During the First World War' in *Journal of the Royal College of Physicians of Edinburgh*, 44:4, 2014 (London: 2014), pp.337–43

Novotny, Jennifer, 'To "take their place among the productive members of society": Vocational rehabilitation of WWI wounded at Erskine' in *Wellcome Open Research*, 2:5, 2017 (London: 2017), pp.1–9

Nunneley, F. P., 'The Whirlpool Bath' in *British Medical Journal*, 25 November 1916 (London: 1916), p.721

12

Scottish Contributions to Surgical Developments in the First World War

Tom Scotland

Henry Gray (1870–1938), John Fraser (1885–1947) and Henry Wade (1876–1955) were three Scottish surgeons who made significant contributions to the management of wounded soldiers in the First World War.

Sir Henry Gray

Henry Gray was born in Aberdeen, the son of a wholesale provision merchant. After leaving school, he began working in his father's business but needed more of a challenge. In 1891 he enrolled to study medicine at the University of Aberdeen, graduating in 1895. He served as a civilian surgeon during the Second Boer War of 1899–1902, but was invalided home after contracting typhoid fever. Thereafter he studied for 18 months in Germany, working in Bonn, Leipzig and Berlin and is credited with the introduction of aseptic surgery to Aberdeen upon his return.[1] He was appointed consultant surgeon to Aberdeen Royal Infirmary in 1904 and soon acquired a reputation as a bold and innovative clinician.

Following the outbreak of war in 1914, Gray was appointed consulting surgeon to a group of base hospitals in Rouen. An evacuation pathway for the wounded had been established in the latter part of the nineteenth century and modified after the Boer War when field hospitals and stretcher bearer companies amalgamated to form field ambulances. The Russo-Japanese War (1904–1905) was associated with many casualties and fearing similar numbers in a European conflict, clearing hospitals were added to the evacuation pathway behind field ambulance facilities which might otherwise

1 Anonymous, 'Obituary, Sir Henry Gray, KBE, FRCS, LLD' in *The Lancet*, 15 October 1938, p.920.

have become overwhelmed. They were renamed casualty clearing stations (CCSs) in January 1915. Definitive surgery in 1914 was delayed until the wounded reached base hospitals near the French coast, a journey that sometimes took days. Penetrating wounds of the chest and abdomen were not considered for operative treatment during the opening months of the conflict, but were kept in clearing hospitals for several days before survivors were evacuated to base hospitals.[2]

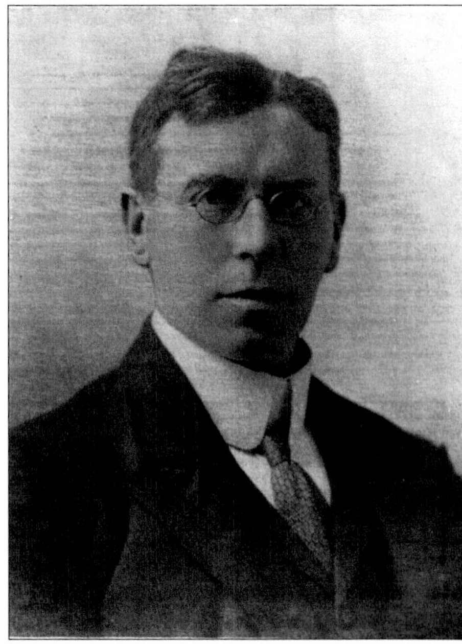

Henry Gray in 1904. (Ann Boyer family archives)

Many wounds in 1914 were regarded as sterile. It was believed that an antiseptic dressing applied to a wound would prevent harmful bacteria gaining access.[3] This regimen was based on experience gained during the Boer War.[4] The latter was fought in dry grasslands of the Transvaal and Orange Free State and most wounds were caused by bullets of relatively low energy fired by Boer marksmen from a considerable distance. Few wounds were caused by shellfire. The Great War in France and Flanders was fought in richly manured fields and the majority of wounds were caused by high explosives, while rifles and machine guns fired sharp-nosed, streamlined bullets of much greater muzzle velocity and destructive power. Fragments of shell casing or bullets drove soiled clothing and debris into wounds along with potentially lethal bacteria. Many wounded reached base hospitals with overwhelming aerobic and anaerobic infections.[5]

The results were appalling. During the first six months of the conflict, the mortality and morbidity from septic wounds dealt to the surgical profession in every nation a staggering blow, from which it recovered only through tedious and painful apprenticeship.[6]

2 Anthony Bowlby, 'The Work of the Clearing Hospitals During the Past Six Weeks' in *British Medical Journal,* 2:2816, 1914 (London: 1914), pp.1053–1054.
3 A. G. Butler, *The Australian Army Medical Services, in the war of 1914–1918,* vol. II (Canberra: Australian War Memorial, 1940), pp.311–312.
4 W. F. Stevenson, *Wounds in War: The Mechanism of their Production and Treatment*, Second Edition (London: Longman Green and Co, 1904). p.130
5 Butler, *The Australian Army Medical Services,* p.312.
6 Butler, *The Australian Army Medical Services,* p.312.

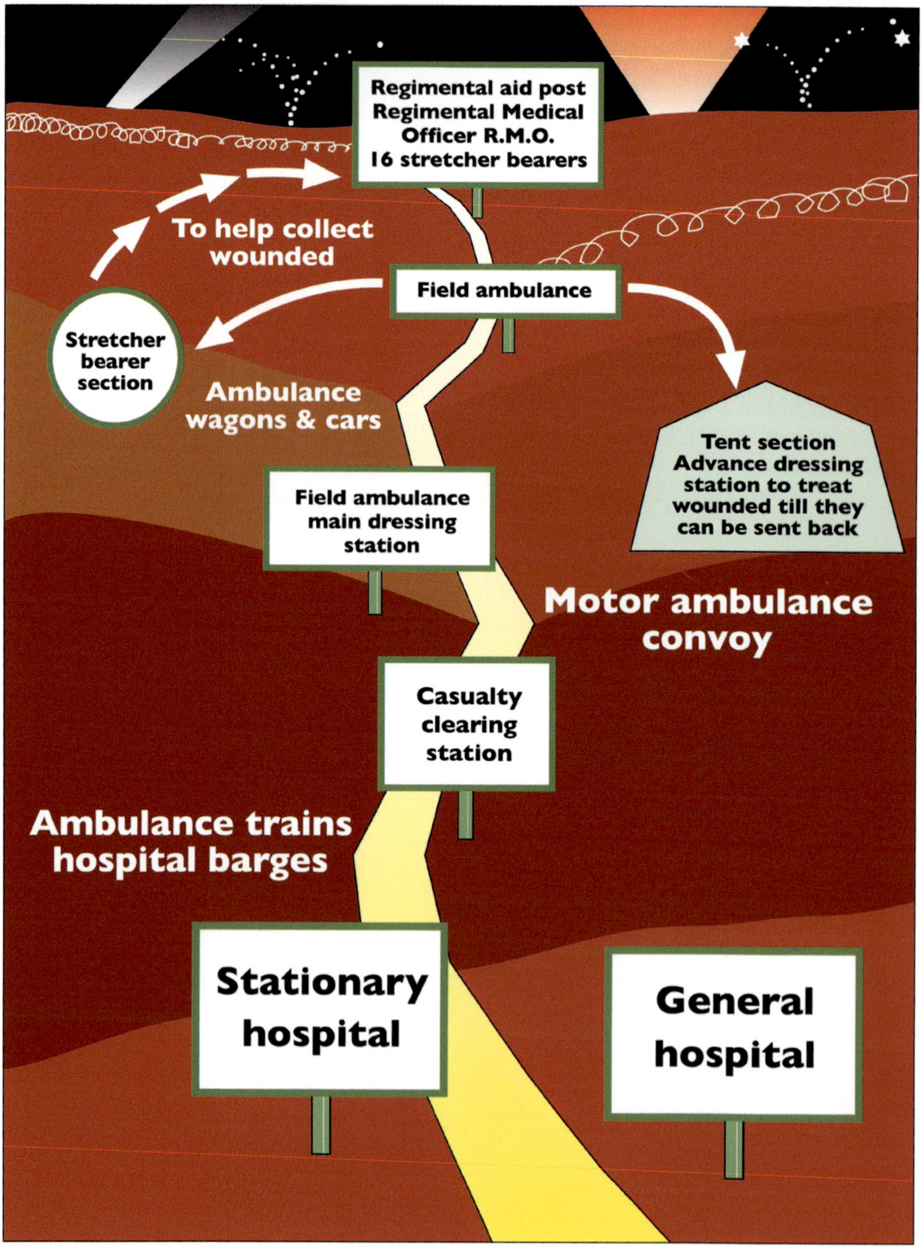

Evacuation pathway for the wounded. (Gordon Stables, Department of Medical Illustration, University of Aberdeen)

Henry Gray and a young Australian Edward Milligan (1886–1972) realised that wounds were contaminated with deadly bacteria from the outset. Antiseptic dressings were useless and early definitive surgery called wound excision was required to remove all necrotic tissue and foreign material, including shell splinters and clothing, converting a filthy wound into a healthy bleeding one. Early surgery was mandatory before infection gained the upper hand. Gray and Milligan described wound excision in June 1915.[7]

Milligan, who was working in a clearing station, faced opposition from surgeons who could not see beyond antiseptic methods of treatment. Fortunately, he had the support of Gray and Sir Anthony Bowlby (1855–1929), the senior British consulting surgeon. Milligan wrote:

> Opposition was so great locally that I first carried out excision of wounds under local anaesthesia, and general anaesthetics induced by myself and continued by an orderly; and this often at late hours and unknown to those in authority. At the request of a consulting surgeon of the army, who opposed this treatment, my commanding officer ordered me to discontinue surgery, and only allowed me to return with the request that I should cease excision of wounds .... Sir Anthony Bowlby, the chief consultant of the B.E.F., expressed himself in agreement with my publication at the time. Sir Henry M. W. Gray, to whom war surgery owes so much, was carrying out the treatment independently at the Base in France, and soon afterwards advocated it energetically at the front.[8]

Patients requiring limb and life-saving surgery were no longer transferred to base hospitals for definitive surgery. It was performed in casualty clearing stations much closer to the front. There were fewer deaths from pyogenic infections and the anaerobic conditions for the gas gangrene organism *Clostridium perfringens* were abolished. The incidence of gas gangrene, which was associated with 25 percent mortality, was reduced from six percent of all wounds to one percent.[9] Gray was very supportive of Milligan, as he was of all young surgeons. He wrote:

> This is a young man`s war, in surgery as well as in purely military matters. The progress of events dictates that younger men should have every chance in a sphere of action where mental and bodily activity count for so much.[10]

7 H. M. W. Gray, 'The Treatment of Gunshot Wounds by Excision and Primary Suture' in *Journal of the Royal Army Medical Corps*, 24: 6, 1915 (London:1915), pp.551–554; E. T. C. Milligan, The early treatment of projectile wounds by excision of the damaged tissue, *British Medical Journal*, 1:2843, 1915 (London: 1915), p.1081.

8 Butler, *The Australian Army Medical Services*, p.328.

9 Butler, *The Australian Army Medical Services*, p.310.

10 H. M. W. Gray, *The Early Treatment of War Wounds* (London: Henry Frowde, Hodder and Stoughton, 1919), p.x.

Sir John Fraser

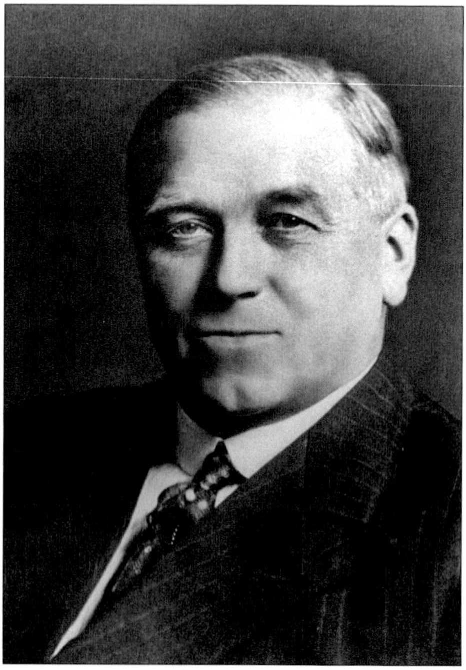

Sir John Fraser in later life. (Collection of Royal College of Surgeons of Edinburgh)

One such young surgeon was John Fraser. Born in Tain in the north of Scotland, he graduated in medicine from the University of Edinburgh in 1907 and established a reputation before the war with outstanding research relating to bone and joint tuberculosis at the Royal Hospital for Sick Children in Edinburgh. He was commissioned Captain in the Royal Army Medical Corps in August 1914 and was appointed regimental medical officer to the 1st Cavalry Division, which fought as infantry with the British Second Army during the final phase of the Second Battle of Ypres in May 1915, at the Battle of Bellewaarde Ridge.[11]

Fraser was transferred to CCS No.7 at Merville in the British First Army sector in northern France where consulting surgeon Cuthbert Wallace was an inspirational figure. Penetrating abdominal wounds in the opening months of the war were treated expectantly in the mistaken belief that soldiers with such wounds fared as well without surgery. The first successful bowel resection was performed by Owen Richards in March 1915.[12] Wallace led an enquiry in May 1915 into the high mortality of penetrating abdominal wounds (80 percent). Most survivors had solid organ involvement. Without surgery, recovery from hollow visceral wounds was very rare. Haemorrhage was the principle cause of early deaths and later deaths were caused by infection. Surgeon General MacPherson ordered the establishment of facilities for the early surgical management of such wounds. During the Battle of Loos (began 25 September 1915), Fraser was put in charge of one advanced operating centre at Bac St Maur, while Richards went to another at Noeux-les-Mines.[13]

Fraser acquired great expertise in the treatment of penetrating abdominal wounds. Timing of surgery was critical. If six hours or less had passed when surgery was

11 J. Graham, 'Sir John Fraser and his Contributions to Surgery' in *Edinburgh Medical Journal*, vol. LVIII: 3, March 1951 (Edinburgh: 1951), pp.105–124.

12 O. Richards, 'The Pathology and Treatment of Gunshot Wounds of the Small Intestine' in *British Medical Journal*, 2:2849, 1915 (London: 1915), pp.213–215.

13 W. G. Macpherson, *History of the Great War based on official documents. Medical Services, General History,* vol. 2 (London: HMSO, 1923), p.457.

performed, the chances were in favour of survival. After six hours, the situation was reversed. A pulse rate of 100 or less carried a good prognosis; 100–120 was associated with an increased mortality and few with a rate greater than 120 survived.[14]

In 1917, Fraser and Hamilton Drummond published a study of three hundred penetrating wounds of the abdomen. Their overall mortality was 56 percent. Their achievement, without the help of penicillin and sulphonamides, with only limited supplies of blood and generally under poor conditions, was remarkable. They emphasised the importance of early surgery with the immediate adequate replacement of blood loss by transfusion of blood or infusion of gum saline; of expeditious operating and of the particular value of colostomy in wounds involving the large bowel.[15]

Shock due to blood loss was a major clinical problem. In August 1917 a Special Investigative Committee on Surgical (wound) Shock and Allied Conditions was established by the Medical Research Committee and chaired by eminent physiologist Ernest Starling (1866–1927). Wound shock was defined as a condition of circulatory failure due to deficient entry of blood into the heart.[16] Fraser was known to be interested and was invited to join. He submitted three studies; on blood pressure changes in wounded soldiers; on the alteration in distribution and character of blood in shock; and on the treatment of shock, including the effect of various intravenous agents.[17] His research was often carried out on or near the front line over two years. He was wounded in 1916 and awarded the Military Cross.

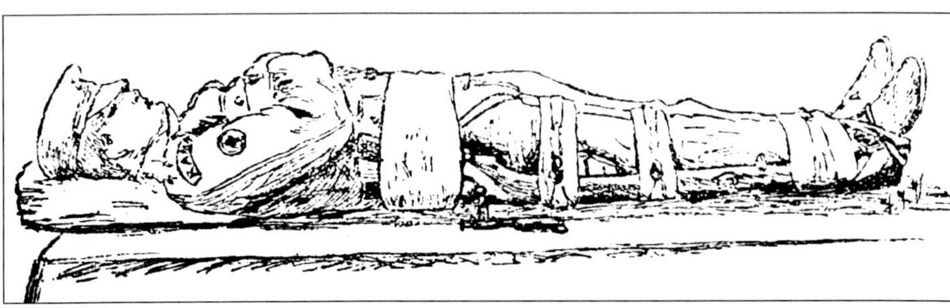

Rifle Splint. (RAMC Handbook 1911)

Fraser also published work on the intravenous use of the antiseptic EUSOL (Edinburgh University Solution of Lime, active ingredients chlorinated lime and

14 C. Wallace, J. Fraser, *Surgery at a Casualty Clearing Station* (London: A & C Black, 1918), pp.157–159.

15 J. Fraser, H. Drummond, 'A Clinical and Experimental Study of Three Hundred Perforating Wounds of the Abdomen' in *British Medical Journal*,1: 2932, 1917 (London: 1917), pp.321–330.

16 Butler, *The Australian Army Medical Services*, p.953.

17 Butler, *The Australian Army Medical Services*, p.953.

boric acid) in patients suffering from toxaemia of gas gangrene, with some apparent success.[18]

The Introduction of the Thomas Splint

Henry Gray was also on the shock committee. Following the Battle of Arras in April 1917, he established a shock centre at CCS No.3 at Gézaincourt, which was a training centre for medical officers and a centre for clinical research. Gray`s interest in shock came partly from experience dealing with compound fractures of the femur (thigh bone), with a documented mortality of 80 percent in 1914 and 1915.[19] The Rifle Splint was standard for femoral fractures in 1914. It failed to adequately immobilise fractures and patients reached CCSs in surgical shock, unable to withstand wound excision to save limbs and lives.

Robert Jones (1857–1933) introduced the Thomas Splint to casualty clearing stations in 1915 and by 1917 Henry Gray was consulting surgeon to the British Third Army under the command of Lieutenant General Sir Edmund Allenby. During the Battle of Arras (6 April–17 May 1917) Gray insisted on the use of the Thomas Splint for femoral fractures. Immobilisation was effective and patients reached designated CCSs in good clinical condition and fit to undergo wound excision. Gray documented a mortality of 15.6 percent in 1,009 cases with an amputation rate of 17.2 percent.[20]

Gray was widely regarded as the leading authority in the management of fractures. Lieutenant Colonel A. D. Carberry, author of the New Zealand Medical History of the Great War, wrote:

> Surgery, especially that of the front line was a specialty of 3rd Army, whose consulting surgeon, Colonel H. M. W. Gray, was noted since 1916 for his work in the treatment of compound gunshot fractures. His memoranda, issued by the Third Army in 1917, formed the basis of the front line surgical practice of this and other armies. His lectures given at Louvencourt were attended by all our medical officers in turn: the problems of shock prevention at the RAP and ADS, the best method of splinting fractures and the demonstration of the regulation set of splints now carried in racks by each motor ambulance, formed the basis of these lectures.[21]

18 J. Fraser & H. Bates, 'Further Observations on the Treatment of Gas Gangrene by the Intravenous Injections of Hypochlorous Acid (EUSOL)' in *British Medical Journal*, 2: 2901, 1916 (London: 1916). pp.172–174.

19 R. Jones, 'Crippling Due to Fractures: its Prevention and Remedy, *British Medical Journal*,1: 3359, 1925 (London: 1925), pp.909–913.

20 Gray, *The Early Treatment of War Wounds*, p.59.

21 A.D. Carberry, *The New Zealand Medical Services in the Great War based on official documents*. (Auckland: Whitcombe and Tombs Ltd., 1924), p.399.

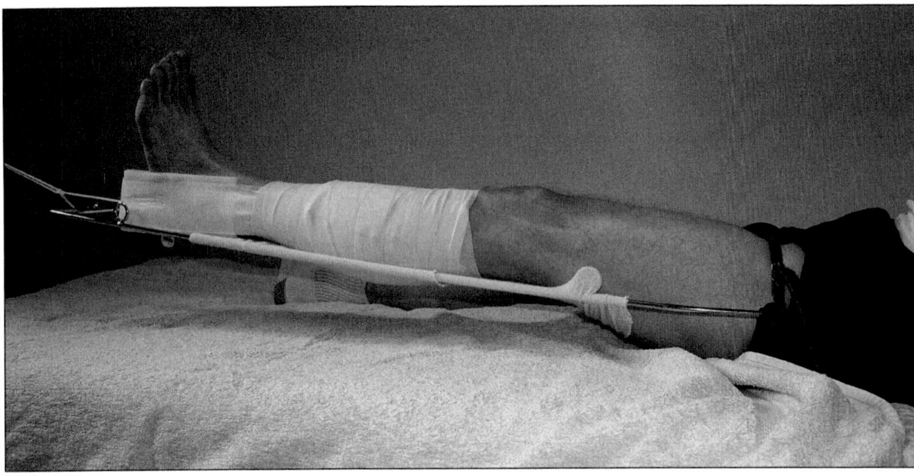

Thomas Splint with skin traction. (Author`s photo)

Henry Gray was one of the most capable surgeons but also one of the most controversial. He was very supportive of young surgeons and in turn was admired by them, but he had a tendency to be intolerant of his contemporaries if they disagreed with him. One, who was a good friend, subsequently wrote of him:

> He had an excellent record and a large personal following among the young surgeons at the front. No man created so much enthusiasm. Henry Gray did the greatest war work at the front, achieving greater practical results than any other surgeon, but his zeal created many enmities among his senior colleagues. A man of his type is necessarily somewhat intolerant of opposition and he may show a want of tact sometimes, for he is essentially a fighter.[22]

One fighter judged to have failed was Lieutenant General Allenby, replaced as commanding officer of the British Third Army when the Battle of Arras ended in stalemate. Lieutenant General Sir Julian Byng took over the Third Army while Allenby was promoted to full General and replaced General Archibald Murray in Egypt in June 1917 as commander of the Egyptian Expeditionary Force, one of whose consulting surgeons was Henry Wade.

22 Diary and letters of Sir Arthur Currie relating to Sir Henry Gray; Archives of McGill University.

Sir Henry Wade

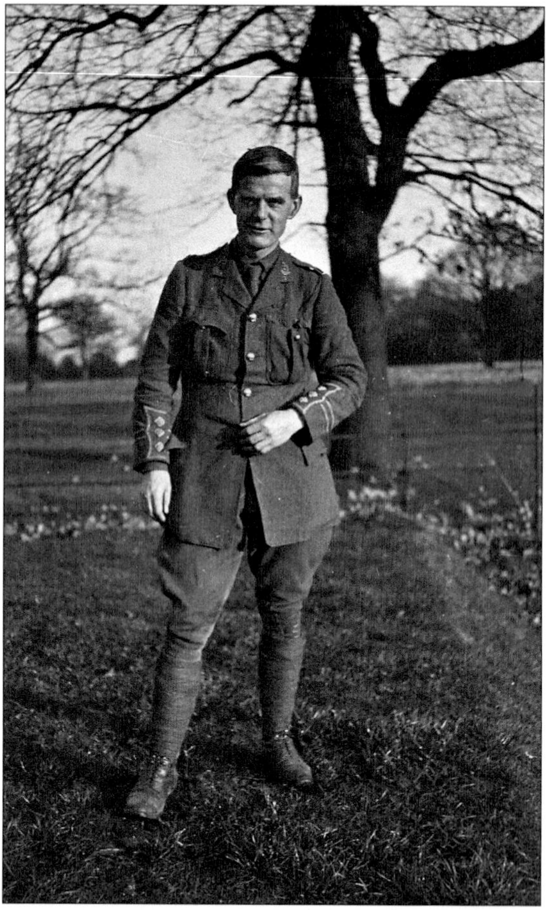

Henry Wade at the park in Blagdon, Northumberland. (Collection of Royal College of Surgeons of Edinburgh)

Henry Wade was born in Falkirk, a son of the Manse. He studied medicine at the University of Edinburgh, graduating with honours in 1898. He served as a volunteer civilian surgeon during the Boer War before returning to Edinburgh to pursue a surgical career. In 1914, he was attached to the Scottish Horse Mounted Brigade Field Ambulance which trained at Morpeth in the north of England. Wade believed that the surgeon should go to the wounded man and not vice versa. He admired French surgeon, Baron Dominique Larrey, who had developed a flying ambulance, an *ambulance volante*, during the Napoleonic Wars. With Larrey's successful endeavours in mind, Wade designed a mobile surgical operation car.[23]

The Scottish Horse Mounted Brigade landed at Gallipoli in September 1915, but there was little scope for Wade`s mobile surgical operation car on the narrow beach with adjacent steep cliff. Contemporary accounts of Wade painted the picture of a man who displayed humanity and humility and who was held in the highest esteem.[24] The Brigade was evacuated to Egypt in December 1915 where Wade became a consulting surgeon to the Egyptian Expeditionary Force in August 1916.

When General Allenby arrived in Egypt, he was instructed to mount an offensive in Palestine and while making preparations, he recalled the very successful Thomas Splint which had been employed during the Battle of Arras. Wade had already been

23 D. Gardner, *Surgeon, Scientist, Soldier; the life and times of Henry Wade 1876–1955* (London: Royal Society of Medicine Press, 1998)

24 Gardner, *Surgeon, Scientist, Soldier*, p.130.

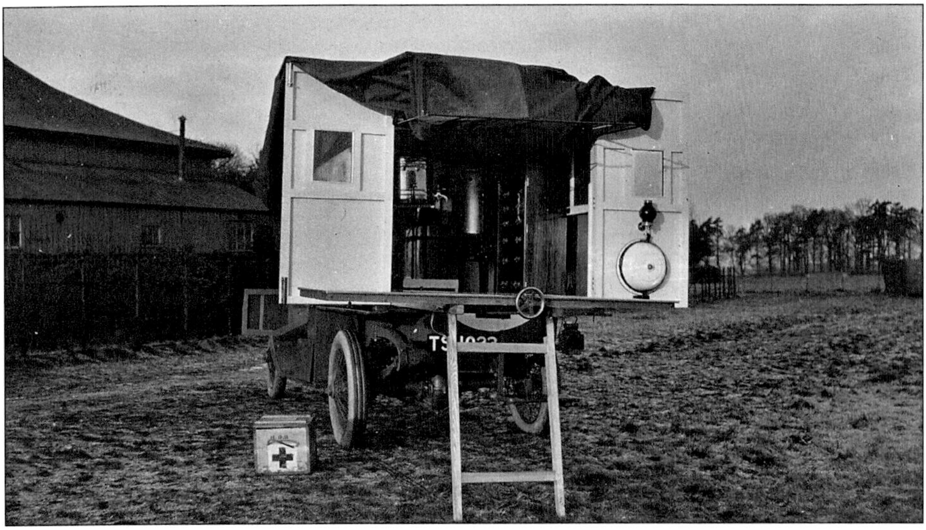

Surgical operation car. (Collection of Royal College of Surgeons, Edinburgh)

advocating its use in Palestine and with Allenby's support, the splint factory in Alexandria made 5,000 Thomas Splints for the coming offensive.

Every general hospital, stationary hospital, casualty clearing station, and field ambulance was encouraged to equip itself with them. The regimental medical officer carried them with his field equipment. The field ambulances had them strapped to their sand carts. Every advanced dressing station was well equipped with them, and a report was called for on any case of this nature that came back from the advanced dressing station without one having been applied.[25]

Beersheba was captured from the Turks on 31 October 1917. A surprise attack by 800 men of the 4th Australian Light Horse Brigade made a significant contribution to the success of this operation. The town and its wells were secured, providing 60,000 allied troops access to the region's only dependable source of water.[26] Gaza was captured on the night of 1/2 November 1917 and Jerusalem was occupied on 9 December 1917. Operations were held up north of Jerusalem for several months, partly due to the transfer of experienced divisions to France to help oppose major German offensives which had begun on 21 March 1918, bringing an end to static warfare on the Western Front. During this delay, malaria in the inhospitable Jordan valley was controlled by draining marshes, depriving the Anopheline mosquito of its breeding ground. An attack north along the coastal plain began on

25 H. Wade, 'Influence of war on the treatment of fractures' in *British Medical Journal*, 1;3140, 1921 (London: 1921), pp.327–330.

26 B. Gardner, *Allenby*, (London: Cassel, 1965), pp.149–150.

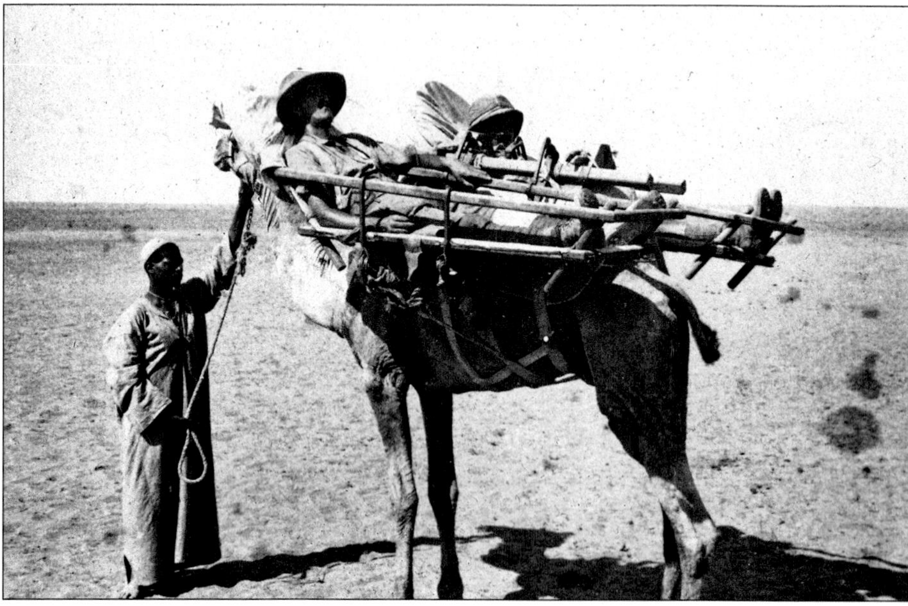

Camel Transport. (Collection of Royal College of Surgeons of Edinburgh)

19 September 1918. Damascus was captured on 1 October 1918 and Aleppo fell on 25 October.[27]

By Western Front standards, distances travelled were great. Damascus was 150 miles from the depots on which the original operation had been based and Aleppo was 200 miles from Damascus. Some advanced units were 200 miles from the nearest railhead, and the main obstacles to the occupation of Syria were distance, supply and disease. Malaria was particularly troublesome and hospital admissions began to rise at an alarming rate just a fortnight after the first breakthrough from Damascus to Aleppo.[28]

Wade had to deal with the problems of distance, supply and disease. He recorded raids deep into enemy territory along virtually non-existent roads. Patients with fractured femurs in Thomas Splints were often transported to the rear by camel for 25 miles to waiting Ford ambulance cars which took the wounded to main dressing stations for definitive surgery, often over wired roads.[29]

Wade stressed the importance of early wound excision and delayed closure. He also recorded that antiseptics were useful for infected cases where definitive treatment

27 A Wavell, *Allenby; A Study in Greatness* (London: George G. Harrap and Co. Ltd., 1940), p.284.
28 Wavell, *Allenby; A Study in Greatness*, p.287.
29 Wade, 'Influence of war on the treatment of fractures'.

had been delayed. He particularly mentioned bismuth iodoform paste and flavine.[30] Wade`s use of antiseptics is reminiscent of the role these agents had during the Boer War, which like the campaign in Palestine was fought in a dry and comparatively sterile environment and where wounds generally healed quickly. This was in stark contrast to appalling conditions in France and Flanders where richly manured fields were contamination by deadly organisms and where reliance on antiseptics in 1914 and early 1915 had proved disastrous.

Epilogue

After the war, Henry Gray returned to Aberdeen, but never settled. He was offered and accepted the position of Chief of Surgery at the Royal Victoria Hospital in Montreal, but his career ended in surgical obscurity when he became the victim of bitter political infighting between the Hospital and McGill University.[31] John Fraser and Henry Wade went back to Edinburgh where their surgical careers flourished and where both men were subsequently honoured in different ways.

Bibliography

Manuscripts

Diary and letters of Sir Arthur Currie relating to Sir Henry Gray; Archives McGill University

Books

Butler, A. G., *The Australian Army Medical Services, in the war of 1914–1918,* Vol. II (Canberra: Australian War Memorial, 1940)

Carberry, A. D., *The New Zealand Medical Services in the Great War based on Official Documents* (Auckland: Whitcombe and Tombs Ltd, 1924)

Gardner, B., *Allenby* (London: Cassel, 1965)

Gardner D., *Surgeon, Scientist, Soldier: The Life and Times of Henry Wade, 1876–1955* (London: Royal Society of Medicine Press, 1998)

Gray, H. M. W., *The Early Treatment of War Wounds* (London: Henry Frowde, Hodder and Stoughton, 1919)

Macpherson, W. G., *History of the Great War based on official documents. Medical Services, General History,* Vol. 2 (London: HMSO, 1923)

Scotland, T. & Boyer, A., *Henry Gray, Surgeon of the Great War: saving lives in a theatre of destruction* (Edinburgh: Capercaillie, 2015)

30 Wade, 'Influence of war on the treatment of fractures'.

31 Scotland, T., Boyer, A., *Henry Gray, Surgeon of the Great War: saving lives in a theatre of destruction* (Edinburgh: Capercaillie, 2015).

Stevenson, W. F., *Wounds in War: The Mechanism of their Production and Treatment*, Second Edition (London: Longman Green and Co, 1904)

Wallace, C., Fraser, J., *Surgery at a Casualty Clearing Station* (London: A & C Black, 1918)

Wavell, A., *Allenby: A Study in Greatness* (London: George G. Harrap and Co. Ltd., 1940)

Journals

Anonymous, 'Obituary, Sir Henry Gray, KBE, FRCS, LLD' in *The Lancet,* 15 October 1938 (London: 1938), p.920

Bowlby, A., 'The Work of the Clearing Hospitals During the Past Six Weeks' in *British Medical Journal,* 2:2816, 1914 (London: 1914), pp.1053–1054

Fraser, J., Bates, H., 'Further Observations on the Treatment of Gas Gangrene by The Intravenous Injections of Hypochlorous Acid (EUSOL)' in, *British Medical Journal,* 2: 2901, 1916 (London: 1916), pp.172–174

Fraser, J., Drummond, H., 'A Clinical and Experimental Study of Three Hundred Perforating Wounds of The Abdomen' in *British Medical Journal*,1: 2932, 1917 (London: 1917), pp.321–330

Gram, J., 'Sir John Fraser and His Contributions to Surgery' in *Edinburgh Medical Journal,* Vol. LVIII: 3, March 1951 (London: 1951), pp.105–124

Gray, H. M. W., The Treatment of Gunshot Wounds by Excision and Primary Suture' in *Journal of the Royal Army Medical Corps,* 24: 6, 1915 (London: 1915), pp 551–554

Jones, R., 'Crippling due to Fractures: Its Prevention and Remedy' in *British Medical Journal,* 1: 3359, 1925 (London: 1925), pp.909–913

Milligan, E. T. C., 'The Early Treatment of Projectile Wounds by Excision of the Damaged Tissue' in *British Medical Journal,* 1:2843, 1915 (London: 1915), p.1081

Richards, O., The Pathology and Treatment of Gunshot Wounds of the Small Intestine' in *British Medical Journal,* 2:2849, 1915 (London: 1915), pp.213–215

Wade, H., 'Influence of War on the Treatment of Fractures' in *British Medical Journa*l, 1:3140, 1921 (London: 1921), pp.327–330

List of Contributors

Iain Macintyre, formerly a surgeon in Edinburgh was Vice President of the Royal College of Surgeons of Edinburgh during its 500th anniversary celebration and served as surgeon to the Queen in Scotland until he retired in 2004. He now writes on the history of medicine and is a past President of the British Society for the History of Medicine.

Michael Crumplin is a retired consultant surgeon, whose prime interest in military conflict is the human aspect of war. He is honorary Curator at the Royal College of Surgeons of England. His four books focus on medicine and surgery, in both the Army and the Royal Navy during the Revolutionary and Napoleonic Wars, 1792–1815. He was education lead for Waterloo200 Project and has donated his medical collection and set up a unique museum of surgery in the farm of Mont St Jean used as the principal field hospital during the Battle of Waterloo in 1815.

Tom Scotland was an orthopaedic surgeon in Aberdeen, who in retirement has developed his longstanding interest in the First World War and the resulting surgical developments. He writes and lectures on the subject and has extended his interest in medical military history to the Napoleonic era with a biography of Sir James McGrigor. He is a member of the Aberdeen Medico-Chirurgical Society, jointly founded by McGrigor.

Peter Brinsden qualified in medicine and then joined the Royal Navy. After gaining the FRCOG he qualified as a Consultant Gynaecologist, retiring in the rank of Surgeon Commander. He was appointed Medical Director of Bourn Hall Clinic, the world's first IVF Clinic. He has four honorary or visiting Professorships from Universities in China, has edited *A Textbook of in vitro Fertilization and Assisted Reproduction,* has published more than 150 peer-reviewed articles and book chapters. He was President of the British Fertility Society, Vice-Chairman of the Nelson Society and is a Fellow of the Royal Geographical Society (FRGS).

Max Cooper is Senior Lecturer in General Practice, at the Brighton and Sussex Medical School. He was a GP in Glasgow and a GP academic fellow at Glasgow

University where he completed his PhD on primary care for asylum seekers. His research interests include the history of medicine, in particular local medical biography from the period of the Napoleonic Wars.

Cat Irving is Human Remains Conservator at Surgeons' Hall Museums, Edinburgh. She has been caring for anatomical and pathological museum collections for over twenty years. At the Royal College of Surgeons of England, she worked with the preparations of William Hunter and then at the Hunterian Museum at Glasgow University. She is a licensed anatomist, and has recently conserved the skeletal remains of the notorious nineteenth century serial killer William Burke. She talks on anatomy and medical history in the UK and abroad. She regularly posts on social media about aspects of medical history in her speciality.

Hilary Morris is an established medical historian, university lecturer, author and journal editor who continues to promote the importance of the history of medicine in both academic and heritage settings. She specialises in nineteenth century British social and military medicine and has researched the development of military and naval preventative health and the colonial impact of cholera.

Peter Starling is a retired RAMC officer who was Curator, and then Director, of the Army Medical Services Museum (now the Museum of Military Medicine) and is now its Honorary President. He lectures on the history of the Army Medical Services and guides battlefield tours in the Far East, Europe and Gallipoli. He holds an MA from the University of Birmingham, a Diploma in the History of Medicine and is a Fellow of the Royal Historical Society.

David Vassallo began his medical education in Malta and completed this at the University of Cambridge, going on to become FRCSEd. He served 35 years with HM Forces in the Royal Army Medical Corps, mainly as consultant general surgeon, retiring in the rank of Colonel. His final post was Military Medical Historian at the Former Army Staff College, during which time he began historical research into the Army Medical Services and took an MA (History of Warfare) at King's College London. He has published four books and several chapters and papers on military medical history topics. He is currently Chairman of Friends of Millbank.

Carol Parry is an archivist by training and is Honorary Librarian at the Trades House of Glasgow. She was formerly the Library and Heritage Manager at the Royal College of Physicians and Surgeons of Glasgow. From 2012–2023 she was Editor of *Scottish Archives*, the journal of the Scottish Records Association, and is a former Secretary of the Scottish Society of the History of Medicine.

Elaine Morrison is a retired Consultant Physician and Rheumatologist. She was the Honorary Librarian at the Royal College of Physicians and Surgeons of Glasgow for two terms and continues as a Senior Fellow. She is currently a member of the Scottish Society of the History of Medicine's Council.

Andreas Demetriades has maintained an interest in the history of medicine alongside his clinical work as Consultant Neurosurgeon in Edinburgh. He has served as Lecturer and Examiner for the Worshipful Society of Apothecaries, run special study modules at the Medical Schools of King's College London and Edinburgh, and is currently President of the Scottish Society of the History of Medicine.

Index